"Rest Ministries, Inc. is a pioneer in acknowledging chronic illness from an emotional and spiritual perspective. The severity of pain is often underestimated in our society, but Lisa Copen genuinely understands pain and how to address it; with education, hope and of course, comfort."

—*Tim Hansel*, author of *You Gotta Keep Dancin'*

So You Want to Start a Chronic Illness Pain Ministry
Copyright © 2001, 2002, by Lisa J. Copen
Cover Design © 2002, JLC Productions

ISBN 0-9716600-0-X

All rights reserved. No part of this book may be reproduced or transmitted in any form or by any means, electronic or mechanical, including photocopying, recording, or any information storage and retrieval system without written permission from Rest Ministries Publishers.

Unless otherwise indicated, all Scripture quotations are taken from the Holy Bible, New International Version. © 1973, 1978, 1984 by International Bible Society. Used by permission of Zondervan Publishing House. All Rights Reserved.

Request for information should be sent to:
Rest Ministries, Inc., a Christian organization
that serves people who live with chronic illness or pain.
P.O. Box 502928, San Diego, CA 92150
858-486-4685; Toll-free 888-751-REST (7378)
Web site: www.restministries.org
Email: rest@restministries.org

Printed in the United States of America

Rest Ministries Publishers

So You Want to Start a Chronic Illness-Pain Ministry

10 Essentials to Make it Work

LISA J. COPEN

Rest Ministries Publishers
SAN DIEGO, CA

Table of Contents

Introduction 7

Chapter 1
Where are all of the chronic illness ministries? 9

Chapter 2
Is there really a need for a chronic illness/pain ministry? 13

Chapter 3
Where is all of the healing? 17

Chapter 4
What exactly is chronic illness/pain ministry? 27

Chapter 5
The etiquette of chronic illness: what to say and what not to say. 41

Chapter 6
Understanding small group ministry: A brief overview 51

Chapter 7
How do I answer their questions about "Why?" 55

Chapter 8
Where do I find resources for my group? 61

Chapter 9
Finding the need and filling it 63

Chapter 10
How to keep the chronic illness/pain ministry in the forefront 71

Introduction

> *"My 9-year-old son and I were in the grocery store when we ran into a woman from our church who stopped me and said, 'Your mother told me you've been having some bad back problems.' I acknowledged that I had. 'Well,' she replied, 'You don't look like you have any problems!' We finished chatting and she left. My son turned to me and said, 'Mommy, how are you supposed to look with your pain?' He had grown up with my dealing with pain almost all of his young life and I didn't let it interfere in my raising him, but he had a pondering question there that I've never forgotten."* — Ellie

There is no doubt that pain hurts. Physical pain is something that most of us will deal with at some point in our lifetimes. Many of us face the unpleasantness of surgeries and accidents, resulting in casts and crutches, followed by an eventual recovery. Chronic pain and chronic illness, however, is never-ending, and it puts those of who live with it in a unique social situation, since we rarely look ill. The invisibility of chronic illness makes it easy to forget about, and the 100+ million people who live with it often have more difficulties dealing with the social and emotional aspects of the illness than learning to cope with the physical pain.

> *"I seriously considered what I could do for vacation bible school, and decided that I should just try to make snacks. A lady who was my age was watching me sign up on the snack sheet, and she chided me, telling me that snacks was what the [elderly] ladies sign up for and that I should be signing up to help with the kids. I know she didn't understand that I have to conserve energy for work, housework, and my family, so I just laughed and signed on the snack sheet. A few months ago when I was still on the steroids, I might have broken down and cried. It's painful to think about how I once was able to do a lot more. Being new at church, where no one knows that, makes it worse."* — Cathy

Unfortunately, when it comes to acknowledging physical pain and chronic illness, the church seems swept up with the rest of society, often becoming blind to this hurting group of people and ignorant in ways in which to minister to them. Often people in pain are searching for answers: "Where is God? How am I going to make it through this? Why is God allowing me to be ill when I've tried to be a good person?" They reach out to their church for answers. Philip Yancey writes in *Where is God When it Hurts?* "The problem of pain is a problem of relationship. Many people want to love God, but cannot see past their tears. They feel hurt and betrayed. Sadly, the church often responds with more confusion than comfort."

Introduction

When a person is ill, the church's response is often to pray for the healing of the person, but when the person is not healed, the church leaders quietly turn away out of frustration and bewilderment. If God chooses not to heal, what more can be done?

This book will help you find the answer to that question.

By reading the countless stories from people who live with illness or pain, you will come to see the need for change in our churches. You will come to see the great need for support from our friends, our peers in Christ.

To make reference easy for you, we have used the following symbols throughout the book.

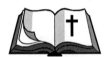

A biblical reference.

Something your church *must* know to be more effective in chronic illness/pain ministry.

You may have picked up this book for a variety of reasons. Perhaps:
- You have a chronic illness.
- Someone you love has a chronic illness
- You want to start a small group/support group at your church.
- You want to teach your church awareness regarding illness.
- You're just curious where disability issues and religion merge.

It is my hope that this book will offer you some background information on spirituality and disability/chronic illness/pain so that you are more aware of how to minister to those who live with chronic illness. It is my prayer that this book will find its way into the hands of someone who has a passion to make a difference, someone who will step forward to lead their church into becoming a refuge for people with chronic illness as the following person has.

> *"I have been talking to my pastor about leading a group such as this and he is all for it. When I was healthy and ministering full-time, I hardly even noticed sick people. Now I can't wait to help them. The Lord has given me a vision!"* – Annie

Lisa Copen
Founder and Executive Director of *Rest Ministries, Inc.*

Chapter 1
Where are all of the chronic illness ministries?

ESSENTIAL #1: Chronic Illness is Invisible
In this chapter you will learn:
- *Why Western medicine has disregarded faith.*
- *Why the church has avoided disability issues.*
- *Why chronic illness/pain ministry is often forgotten.*

So, you want to start a chronic illness ministry! The logical first step would be to look around for other chronic illness/pain support groups that are in churches, and see how they are functioning. You may be surprised, however, to find that there is not an abundance of these groups and that most churches have never thought of starting such a group. Why are there so few illness/pain groups with a Christian slant that embrace the issues of living with a chronic condition?

Historically, disability and ministry are no strangers. Religious and charitable societies have always assisted the disabled with humane care and financial support. Even in the world of academia, the study of disability/illness and religion has not been adequately researched. These are a few comments from those who have written articles for *The Disability Quarterly*.

- "Disability within diverse religious, cultural, and historical contexts have only very recently begun to be explored" (1).
- "Religious stories of people with disabilities... are a largely untapped resource for researchers" (2).
- "Historically, the experience of people with disabilities has been an untapped source for theology, often even theology related to disability" (3).
- "The impact of religion and spirituality in the lives of people with disabilities and their family members has been insufficiently investigated" (4).

With the academic world declining an interest or deeming this combination of topics "unnecessary," is it any surprise that the media and our resources hesitate to publish books on the subject, write magazine articles, and establish such ministries? Let's take a closer look at why there is a shortage of chronic illness/pain ministries.

Western Medicine has Disregarded Faith
It comes as no surprise that the medical establishment has its own sense of values, and it is rarely interested in expanding those values to include the opinions of religious professionals and patients. "Religious professionals

Chapter 1

have not always been allowed to evaluate the spiritual needs of people in crisis, much less minister to these needs," writes Blair and Blair in *Pastoral Counselors/Religious Professionals and People with Disabilities*. "This has begun to change as spiritual strength and the power of faith become more apparent as aids in healing, but it is still not uncommon for the spiritual counsel to be ignored altogether or, at best, consulted as an afterthought."

There have been gradual changes in this attitude as organizations like the International Center for the Integration of Health and Spirituality (formerly the National Institute of Health Research), have taken strides in researching the relationship between spirituality and health. The late Dr. David Larson, former president of NIHR co-authored the article "Religion and Spirituality in Medicine: Research and Education" that appeared in the September 3, 1997 issue of the *Journal of the American Medical Association*. The article emphasizes how research has shown that doctors should start paying more attention to spiritual issues and the spirituality of their patients. Dr. Larson said, "Reporting these findings in a respected journal like *JAMA* sends physicians a message that religion is a health factor that they need to take seriously." It has taken a long time to get to this point, but faith is beginning to be recognized in the medical arena.

▶ Does this mean that the doctors across the country are asking their patients to join them in prayer? *It's unlikely.*

▶ Do these changes signify that your doctor will be more tolerant of your religious beliefs? *Very possibly.*

▶ Will this research see the emergence of health ministries and chronic illness/pain ministries? *We have yet to find out.*

The Church has Avoided Disability Issues

The church has been involved with the disabled community for centuries, and yet only recently has the disabled community been able to emerge and speak for themselves. In the past, due to a variety of assumptions, the disabled population was given little intellectual credibility, and others spoke "about them" (not for them).

Although churches may have good intentions when it comes to ministering to those who live with illness or disability, the church body is made up of individuals who are influenced by society and our social culture. It is only natural that these individuals cope with circumstances in human ways which may not always be tactful or even spiritually correct.

> *"I have had eight major back surgeries over the past 12 years with various knee blow-outs and hernias. I have traveled the church wilderness and more often then not was condemned by well-meaning believers who did not know*

> *His Word. People tend to believe that the bible says God wants this flesh to be comfortable and have everything it desires. I could not find this translation."* — Willie

> *"I have used a wheelchair for eighteen years. What does it mean to the average person to encounter me? Whatever else it may mean, it is to be reminded of his/her own vulnerability and the vulnerability of those whom they love. To be reminded, at however deep a level, that they and theirs are but a traffic accident, a fall, a dive into a too-shallow pool away from being — in their language — a cripple, or, worse yet, a 'helpless cripple.' To be reminded that even in their sleep in the safety of their homes, a sinister disease can creep in and begin chewing away at nerve and muscle tissue, undetected until it is too late. They see me as loss, as option no longer available, as life's hopes and dreams aborted. Life as existing, not flourishing. And ultimately, as a harbinger of their own final vulnerability, death"* (Betenbaugh).

Let's face it: none of us like to be reminded of our vulnerability. It's easier for us to believe that the person who has an illness or disability must have it for a reason. God is a loving God who is all-powerful, so He would not allow this person to suffer unless there was a reason, right? It is easier for us to reassure ourselves, "Perhaps that person has unconfessed sin in her life, and that is why she is suffering." Then we realize that we too have some sin in our own lives that we have been trying to avoid confronting, and we begin to fear that God will punish us too.

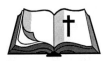

These fears aren't all that unusual. Even Job's friends felt this way when they saw the destruction that God was bringing into Job's life. They knew that Job had been a faithful servant to God, and yet they saw his life being devastated. So what was their response? They condemned Job and told him it was his own fault and that he should just repent so he could get on with life. Job's friend, Eliphaz, said, "Consider now: Who, being innocent, has ever perished? Where were the upright ever destroyed? As I have observed, those who plow evil and those who sow trouble, reap it. We have examined this, and it is true. So hear it and apply it to yourself," (Job 4:7-8;26,27).

Regardless of the array of emotions we feel, one thing is certain: It's very common to feel awkward fellowshipping with an ill person. She may remind us of our own vulnerability in this imperfect world. She may remind us of our own sin. Seeing her suffer makes us question the wisdom of the God, in whom we put our faith; that He would allow such circumstances to befall us or the ones we love.

So, does the church organize a ministry for these people who live with pain and need support and encouragement from one another? So far, the answer has been, not likely. We are hoping that this is about to change.

Why is Chronic Illness/Pain Ministry Forgotten?

Support groups have become places of refuge for people in the last fifteen years, and churches have recognized that people have a deep desire to share

Chapter 1

not only their emotional struggles, but also the spiritual struggles they have along their journey of recovery. Whether it's called a small group, support group or care group, churches have been taking steps to address these needs by offering supportive groups within the church community. People who live with issues of alcoholism, eating disorders, sexual abuse, divorce recovery, blended families and addiction are able to find a supportive, nurturing environment. With attendance, and sometimes repentance, one can be healed and enjoy the fellowship of others. So where are all of the chronic illness ministries?

Did you see that key word in the description of groups? *Heal.* Many people are attending these groups in order to be healed. Whether it be an emotional, a mental, a spiritual healing or all three, each person comes seeking healing. If you are wondering why there aren't enough chronic illness/pain support groups, one reason is this: when churches and other organizations try to minister to the ill, the focus is often that of physical healing, not necessarily the emotional healing.

When the prayers for a physical healing are not answered, then what? Elders and others oftentimes dismiss the unanswered prayer as a sign from God that one of the following has occurred.
- The person with the illness lacked faith.
- The person with the illness has unconfessed sin in his or her life.
- The person with the illness has not asked for forgiveness.
- The prayer was not done correctly.
- Someone who prayed lacked faith.

Unfortunately, the person who needs the most support and encouragement is often left feeling condemned and even more isolated than before she was prayed for. If God doesn't care about her, and people in the church are judgmental, where can she turn?

She can turn to *a HopeKeepers (TM)* small group, a refuge for people who want to live, not just survive, with chronic illness.

But who wants to lead a group of people who have gone through such an experience? Who amongst us feels qualified to lead such a group? Who of us can explain to a person why God is not healing her? Does the leader of a chronic illness small group pray for healing or help? Function or faith? Answered prayer or patience? Keep on reading! You may be surprised to find yourself saying, "I could do this!" or "This just may work."

1　Whyte, 1995, Turner, 1984 in "Religion and Disability Studies: Thoughts on Status and Future of an Emerging Dialogue." Eieslane, Nancy, L. Ph.D., Assistant Professor, Sociology of Religion, Candler School of Theology, Emory University, Atlanta, GA. in *Disability Studies Quarterly*, Summer 1995, Volume 15, No. 3.
2　Fontaine, 1995 "Religion and Disability Studies: Thoughts on Status and Future of an Emerging Dialogue." Eieslane, Nancy, L. Ph.D., Assistant Professor, Sociology of Religion, Candler School of Theology, Emory University, Atlanta, GA. in *Disability Studies Quarterly*, Summer 1995, Volume 15, No. 3.
3　Ibid.
4　Enteen, Ph. D. "Religion , Spirituality and Disability: A Health Services Research Agenda" in *Disability Studies Quarterly*, Summer 1995, Volume 15, No. 3.
5　Dr. David Larson. "Religion and Spirituality in Medicine: Research and Education" in *The Journal of the American Medical Association*, September 3, 1997.

Chapter 2
Is there really a need for chronic illness/pain ministry?

ESSENTIAL #2: Chronic Illness Ministry is Needed
In this chapter you will learn:
- Why there is a need for chronic illness/pain ministry.
- Why pastoral counseling isn't enough.
- Why a secular support group isn't enough.

"There Aren't that Many People in Our Church Who Have a Chronic Illness"

You may ask yourself, "Is there really a need for this kind of ministry at my church?" Are people calling the office to see if you have a pain ministry? Probably not. Do you see people who are hurting and wonder if they would like some support? No. Do people come forward at your service and ask for prayer when they have been diagnosed with an illness? Yes, they do. "But they ask for healing" you reply. "Not to get together with other people and talk about it." You're right. Despite the fact that over 100 million people are living with chronic illness, we don't seem to notice them. We don't see their pain. Why is this?

> *"I used to go to church all of the time. It gradually became hard to sit through the service. My legs would get stiff, and so I couldn't just stand up and walk out gracefully and quietly. So I missed a few weeks and no one seemed to notice. Eventually, I just quit going. I try to have a quiet time now and then and I still believe in God and all of that, but my relationship with God has really faltered. I just felt like none of those people at my church really understood, and they were my last hope."* – Sarah

Despite what you may think, there are *many* people who live with invisible chronic illness who are attending your church right now. If you could take your church, turn it upside down and shake it so all of the people who live with invisible chronic illness fell out, you would lose entire pews...maybe half the choir. Don't be surprised if your pastor and a handful of children are included.

> *"One of the hardest things for me is that I do not look disabled at all. I have a terminal illness, but my body appears healthy from the outside at this stage of my disease. People cannot see anemia when you wear make-up. They cannot see my malignant hypertension. They do not know I have had four major surgeries on my head. They just say, 'Oh, what lovely blond hair you have!'"* – Jenny

Chapter 2

"We all Have a 'Cross to Bear.' Do The Chronically Ill Really Need a Ministry?"

Chronic illness and disability are often not seen as their own entity of suffering. Although our Christian bookstores now have shelves stocked full of books on life's problems that we may encounter, chronic illness is simply seen as a form of suffering, and therefore, is often seen as something that does not need to be specifically addressed. Since the Middle Ages, Christianity has viewed impairments or physical ailments as indistinguishable from other forms of suffering. Susan Reynolds Whyte, author of *Disability Between Discourse and Experience* (1), writes "Infirmity [impairment] and poverty were part of God's varied creation—the order of things. The response to difference was charity, spirituality, and morality."

There are many excellent books written by Christians on the topic of suffering, and a chronically ill person will likely find some comfort in them. We all wish to be able to identify, however, with the specific circumstances. Sometimes we need illness to be addressed specifically, especially since it brings out so much confusion with regard to faith and spirituality. Who among us would not enjoy picking up a book that described what we are feeling and gave us the sense that we are not alone in our struggles?

> *"I got your newsletter and sat down on the couch to read it right away. As soon as I started to read the front page, I started to cry because you explained exactly how I had been feeling the last week, but had been unable to express. I felt such a sense of relief knowing I wasn't alone. My husband walked in and saw my tears and said, 'What's wrong?' and then I had him read it too and he cried with me. Thank you for this gift."*
> -a subscriber of ...And He Will Give You Rest *newsletter*

None of us like to feel that we are alone in our experience. Discarding the pain and the emotional and spiritual upheaval that illness brings into our life as merely "suffering" is not acceptable. We are aware that life is not going to be easy. We are warned in 1 Peter 4:12 "Do not be surprised at the painful trial you are suffering, as though something strange were happening to you," but we still want someone there beside us.

Isn't This What A Pastor is For?

Surprisingly, most pastors do not receive specific training for chronic illness/disability ministry. Many of them will come to understand what to say and how to respond out of experience. You may ask, "If the pastor isn't even addressing this issue, does it really need to be addressed?" The answer is, of course, yes. "Religion serves ordinary people who have

> *Looking at a variety of illnesses from cardiovascular conditions to cancer, researchers found that frequent attendance at worship services was linked to healthier lives.*(2)

accidents and diseases, who bear children with congenital conditions and develop heart problems, arthritis, and much more in maturity," says Blair and Blair, authors of *Pastoral Counselors/Religious Professionals and People with Disabilities* (3). "Life is change, not always for the better. And very often the parish minister will be the spiritual helper to whom people will turn."

When a people are diagnosed with a chronic illness, it affects their entire being, especially their spirituality. Even the person who may claim to be an atheist is suddenly asking, "Why me, God?" When a person is diagnosed with a permanent disability or a chronic illness, many well-meaning pastors are at a loss as to how to explain why the person is going through what he or she is going through. The person is dealing with a wide array of emotions.

They :
- doubt themselves
- doubt the existence of God
- blame themselves
- blame God

They are filled with:
- fear
- anger
- bitterness
- depression

Blair and Blair state "This is the time of greatest need, as well as a time when spiritual and physical suffering coexist in its rawest form. People have their spiritual advisors label them as sinners, question their faith, chastise them for feeling angry, tell them they were 'chosen by God' to be 'an inspiration,' and avoid any discussion of the dramatic life changes these people and their families are facing."

"Support for people with disabilities and their families can mean the survival of the family unit, and the most effective religious professionals know what support is needed and where to find it," writes Blair and Blair. "It is not unusual for families to consult a minister for advice about counseling, effective support groups, shared care programs, and sources of economic aid."

"Can't They Just Go to a Secular Support Group?"

There is no doubt that support groups are beneficial. Stanford Medical School researchers recently found that women with metastatic breast cancer (cancer that had spread to other organs or their bones) survived longer if they were part of a support group led by a psychiatrist or social worker along with a therapist who had breast cancer in remission. Five years after the study began, the data showed that women who became part of a support group lived twice as long as the women who did not participate, which surprised the study's lead scientist, David Spiegel, who had set out to *disprove* the idea that psychosocial interventions could prolong life. (4)

This said, support groups don't meet all of our needs. Whether a person is seeking to express his anger at God or seeking for the support of God, he is oftentimes discouraged from expressing these thoughts at secular group meetings. It is common to leave the meetings feeling as though something is missing. Oftentimes, these meetings focus on the education of one's illness and how to live a productive life despite the limitations. The facilitators try to come up with positive agendas for the meetings, but ultimately, the only hope that is given is hope for a cure or a more effective drug.

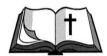

Although a cure or more effective drug would be nice, as Christians, we don't need to put our ultimate hope in these things, because we have a hope in God. Our hope lies in things unseen. Hebrews 11: 1 says "Faith is being sure of what we hope for and certain of what we do not see." When a faith-centered support group meets, we can always leave with a hope that is not of this world; a hope that regardless of what lies ahead in the medical world, we have a better world that we will one day be a part of: heaven. Our hope can be our anchor for our soul, firm and secure and hope will not be cut off, (Proverbs 23:18).

> *"I need a place to talk about the spiritual aspect of living with a chronic illness; a group of people who are a refuge; people who understand what it's like to deal with pain every day. I feel that the spiritual journey one takes when she is diagnosed with a chronic illness is an important part of how she copes and lives out her life."* – Patti

Friendships with other Christians who are experiencing similar challenges, frustrations, and even lessons are a vital part of one's emotional well-being. Though "even in laughter the heart may ache," (Proverbs 14:12b), most of us who live with chronic illness or pain will agree that there is nothing that can replace friendships with other Christians who understand our journey.

---

1 Susan Reynolds Whyte. "Disability Between Discourse and Experience" in *Disability Studies Quarterly*, Summer 1995, Volume 15, No. 3.
2 Levin, J.S. and Vanderpool, H. Y. "Is Frequent Religious Attendance Really Conducive to Better Health? Toward an Epidemilogy of Religion." *Social Science and Medicine*; 247(7):589-600.
3 Blair and Blair. "Pastoral Counselors/Religious Professionals and People with Disabilities" in *Disability Studies Quarterly*, Summer 1995, Volume 15, No. 3.
4 "Effect of Psychosocial Treatment on Survival of Patients with Metastatic Breast Cancer" by Speigel, D, J. R. Bloom, H. C. Kraemer, & Gottheil, E., *The Lancet*, 8668, 2, 1989, pp. 888-891.

Chapter 3
Where is all of the healing?

ESSENTIAL #3: *Healing is a Personal Issue*
In this chapter you will learn:
- Why healing is a personal issue.
- Why prayer for healing should not be done out of obligation or cohersion.
- Why healing does not necessarily signify a hidden sin or a lack of faith.
- Why it's important to understand that God's healing is not always a physical thing.

God can heal. God is capable of taking a person out of the depths of life-threatening illness to wellness in a mere moment. So why doesn't He? Why doesn't He heal more people? Even more of a mystery, why doesn't He at least heal good, faithful servants who have faith that God will heal them?

Unfortunately, you won't find the answers to these questions in this book, but these issues, mysteries, and how to answer others who are asking these questions will be addressed.

There are a lot of assumptions about healing:
- everyone who is a "good Christian" will be healed.
- God wants everyone to be healed of physical ailments.
- everyone who has an illness wants to be prayed over for healing.
- those who have enough faith will be healed.
- everyone should want to be healed.
- saying "I will pray for you to be healed" is always the right thing to say.
- reassuring someone, "I know God will heal you" is acceptable.

This chapter includes a lot of first-person accounts, because healing is a very personal issue. Only by asking how people feel about healing and putting our assumptions aside can we begin to understand.

Healing is a Personal Issue

"There are some people in my small group who are able to see the subtle clues in my body language and face that I'm in pain, and who will ask me if I'd like to pray. They really ask me, not ask having already made up their mind what it is that I need for them to do." – Sherry

"Disabled people are healed in miracle stories," says Hurst, author of *Disability From the Point of View of Religion and Spirituality* (1). "These are often taken literally to mean that all disabled people should and would want to be healed in this way." In John 5:6 Jesus asks a man who has been an invalid for thirty-eight years "Do you want to be healed?" Most of us may ask, "What kind of a question is that? Who would not want to be healed?"

Upon hearing many people's experiences about being prayed over for healing, there was one underlying theme. People want to be *asked*. This may come as a surprise to those who do not live with physical ailments, because the desire to be healed seems to be assumed. Over and over, people shared, however, that they resented people assuming that they wanted prayer for healing and that they appreciated people asking, "What would you like me to pray for?" Surely, Jesus understood this.

> *"People have prayed for me for healing when I did not want it, and it has led me to feel uncomfortable with continued pain. I do not feel it is acceptable to remind people of this recurring need. I have also chosen to have prayer for healing from pain, because I felt the need, and the pain was relieved--as was the emotional distress I had been feeling."* – Cheri

Throughout the bible, Jesus heals numerous people, but many of them came to Jesus asking for healing. When Jesus approached the man at the pools, the man may have even believed that Jesus was being sarcastic with him. "Who is this guy messing with me about healing? All I want to do is get into the pools, but people keep getting in front of me! Can he do something about that? Now *that* would be helpful!" The man had been an invalid for thirty-eight years, and when Jesus asked him "Do you want to get well?" the man didn't even answer Jesus' question, possibly believing that Jesus obviously didn't understand the circumstances.

Although we may know that God can heal us, when we live with illness or disability, we often feel that healing is a personal thing between ourselves and God. When people assume we want to be prayed for, despite their loving intentions, it is a sign of disrespect. It makes those of us with illness feel foolish, as though we haven't considered that God can heal us with the swoop of His hand.

> *"When I was recently in much constant pain and having months of sleepless nights due to pain and other things, I was put on the prayer list in the bulletin without my knowledge. At first, it bothered me. I usually keep this just within a few close friends so that I don't have to do a lot of explaining of the problem."* – Ellie

This is a difficult thing for a church to understand. It should be standard practice, however, for anyone in leadership (or not) who is in a situation where a prayer for healing is believed to be desired, the person to be prayed over should be asked, "Would you like me/us to pray for your healing?" Or one can ask the person, "What would you like us to pray for?" Don't assume the answer is obvious. Many people will respond, "Please pray for my healing," and then one can be rest assured that the person feels comfortable asking God for healing.

Other people may respond to this question by saying, "Pray for God to give me the strength to get through this" or "Pray that I can accept God's will." Although it may be tempting to slip in the words "God, please heal this person's body" this shows a sign of disrespect, and that will send up red flags to the ill person that you don't understand, nor do you care to understand. To truly give the person comfort and peace, pray for what they ask you to pray for.

How do you pray for a person who doesn't request healing? Here are some things that you can pray for:
- Say, "Lord, we don't even know what to ask for, but we know that You know our hearts."
- Ask God to bring the ill person comfort.
- Ask God to end or decrease the pain.
- Ask God to bless him with good rest and sleep.
- Ask God to give wisdom and discernment in the medical decisions that need to be made.
- Ask God to be with the ill person's family and loved ones who are worried.
- Ask God to be with the ill person's children who may be staying somewhere other than their own home.
- Ask God to give the doctors wisdom and discernment.
- Ask God to bring good caregivers/nurses into the person's environment.
- Ask God to send friends into the ill person's life.
- Ask God for effective medications with few side effects.

David Beibel shares this story in his book *How to Help a Heartbroken Friend* (2).
> "When Naomi was eighteen months old, spinal meningitis stole the hearing in her right ear. Three days after Christmas 1987, at forty-five years of age, she woke up to find herself totally deaf from the delayed effect of the same disease. What hindered her recovery most was not all the lifestyle adjustments required, though these were formidable enough, but 'those who insisted that by going to some healing service I would be miraculously healed—or the pastor -'friend' who wanted to pray for revelation of something in my past that was hindering my healing,' Naomi wrote. 'They looked on it as temporary testing by God and said we just needed to pray the right way. At the same time I was trying to accept the permanence of it. I do believe some are healed miraculously, but I felt I was not one of them, and to keep insisting that I go to some prayer meeting so they could pray for me was hindering the grief process. They were not accepting what I was trying accept." (page 61).

Prayer for Healing Should Not be Done Out of Obligation

"I was healed of two incurable illnesses, but it does not seem to be in God's plan at present to heal me of chronic fatigue syndrome. I've been in prayer groups where you felt an obligation, and I resented that immensely."
– Virginia

Chapter 3

We all have a great desire to see our friends and family well. Who of us wants to see someone we love suffer? Circumstances are rarely in our control, however, and as Christians, what is the first thing we tend to do when things are beyond our control? We pray about it! We pray that God will right the wrongs, correct the crooked, and heal the sick. It's easy to get caught up in the excitement of seeing God work.

> *"I think the worst thing is when people want to pray for complete healing of my pain and/or disability. Sometimes I get the impression that if this doesn't happen they feel something is wrong with me or their prayer. That it's not okay to be in pain or to suffer, not really and truly. That God would never want us to continue to be in pain...which is, of course, not what God says in the Bible at all!!"* – Cherie

Enthusiasm about healing is not always contagious, and healthy people can't understand why an ill person isn't excited about the potential to see God work in his or her life. We insist on praying for them. We insist on dumping oil on their head, and we impatiently wait for God to "zap 'em!" We want to hear God first hand say "Pick up your mat and walk," (John 5:11), "Take off the grave clothes and let him go," (John 11:44), "Woman, you are set free from your infirmity," (Luke 13:12). We may get so excited about the healing, however, that we forget about the person.

> *"I have been prayed for several times. Finally, I asked Him myself and I heard a resounding, 'no.' It's time to move on and somehow make this a positive experience."* – Rebecca

There are a variety of reasons why an ill person may not wish to have someone pray for her healing. Some of these are positive, acceptable reasons. Others are understandable, but not spiritually correct. Either way, a person should *never* be forced, coherced, or obligated to be prayed over. You can always pray silently; God hears us regardless.

Some of the positive reasons may include:
- She feels like God is blessing her through the illness.
- She has come to view the world differently since she was diagnosed.
- She has come to know God on a deeper level because of her illness.
- She may worry about what would happen to her faith if she didn't have to depend on God as much as she does now while living with this illness.
- She is seeing God work through her illness and use it to help other people.

There is a wide variety of ways that churches go about praying for healing. Some have altar calls or revivals. Others have the ill person come to the church office and quietly be prayed for by the elders. Regardless of how your church does it, it is important that the ill person and their comfort zone be respected. A church or leaders within the church should never insist on praying for someone out loud if the person does not want to be prayed for (and if she is asked, you will know!) If the person feels uncomfortable, the church risks that person never returning or returning but never feeling comfortable in that church again.

"Rosalie visits a church for the first time. Because she is deaf, but can do pretty well with her hearing aids, she sits in the front. When the healing service begins, she is asked to come forward. Feeling pressured, she does. The minister prays loudly, covers her ears, and asks the Lord to heal her. She is stunned, but wants to be polite. The next week, when she visits the church again, she leaves her hearing aids off. Now Rosalie can understand almost nothing, but she does not want to disappoint all of the people who prayed for her," (3).

Some of the understandable, but spiritually incorrect reasons a person does not want anyone to pray for their healing may include:
- She doesn't believe that God is concerned enough about her to heal her.
- She doesn't think that she has enough faith in God to be healed.
- She thinks that the illness is her punishment and she deserves it.
- She believes that she has committed too many sins to ask for God to heal her.

If one feels these are the reasons that a person refuses prayer for healing, then a minister or even a good friend should counsel this person on what it means to be a Christian. The person may need to be led into accepting Jesus Christ, asking for forgiveness and understanding God's grace. Under these circumstances, however, it is important that the person understand that healing is not guaranteed just because she has become a Christian. Whether one is healed or not is not dependent on good works, the amount of faith, or sin which has been confessed. She will likely have many questions, and a chronic illness/pain small group would be a good place for her to gain insight and emotional support.

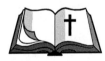

Lack of Healing Does Not Necessarily Signify a Hidden Sin

> *"When I was at an intercessory prayer meeting to pray for the church, everyone decided to pray for me. They tried to get me to confess my 'hidden sin,' saying that I was hiding something. After six years of suffering with a terminal illness, I had and have confessed all that I know as sin, and I have come to realize that His grace is sufficient for me. I am hiding no 'hidden sin.' I am very transparent and can honestly say that there is not one day that goes by where my holiness will ever stack up. I am either saved by the blood of Jesus or I am not."* – Jenny

When Jesus heard that his good friend Lazarus was ill, he responded by saying, "This sickness will not end in death. No, it is for God's glory so that God's Son may be glorified through it," (John 11:4). Jesus didn't say, "He is ill because of sin." There are instances in the Bible where a warning is given. When Jesus healed the man by the pools He then told him, "Stop sinning or something worse may happen to you," (John 5:14). The man did have sin in his life, but Jesus chose to approach the man and offer him healing despite the sin.

From this, can we assume that not all illness is a result of sin? And even if there is sin, Jesus still has the option to heal us in spite of it. When a person prays for healing and is not healed, oftentimes the people around him will quickly assume

Chapter 3

that the person has sin in his life and that is why God has refused to heal. This way, God is understandable to us. We who do not live with physical limitations can rest easy that nothing will happen to us since we are obeying God.

God doesn't work this way. As mentioned earlier, his ways are different that our ways. We cannot comprehend how he chooses to make decisions. When we try to package him into a box and say, "'A' plus 'B', must equal 'C,'" we are limiting the greatest power and making judgements where we have no knowledge.

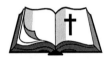

Lack of Healing Does Not Necessarily Signify a Lack of Faith

"Rise and go. Your faith has made you well," (Luke 17:19). There are various incidents throughout the Bible where the Word refers to one being healed because of his or her faith. When a woman approached Jesus, sure that by just touching His clothing she would be cured her from her sickness, Jesus responded by saying, "Daughter, your faith has healed you. Go in peace and be freed from your suffering."

Does this mean that when one is not healed it is because of a lack of his or her faith? Oftentimes, when healing does not occur people are quick to say, "You weren't healed because you did not have enough faith." Is all healing dependent on faith?

> *"We don't know the hearts of those who aren't healed, only God does. But oftentimes I've seen people who weren't healed under condemnation when the pain doesn't lift. There is truth involved with a lot of damaging condemnation. This is hurtful and painful to hear." – Kathy*

According to Mark 6:5,6, it is possible to be healed even when there is a lack of faith present. "He (Jesus) could not do any miracles there, except lay his hands on a few sick people and heal them. And He was amazed at their lack of faith."

These people in Jesus' hometown lacked faith—so much so that even Jesus was amazed, yet He chose to have compassion on them and heal them anyway. Who are we to judge why a person has not been healed? Only our Lord can truly know why He has not chosen (or has chosen) to heal a person.

> *"At my church, I have been meeting with a prayer counselor, in this case the Minister of Counseling and her prayer partner. They 'soak' me in prayer. It is a time of being ministered by the spirit and a reminder that God is holding us, even through this illness. We also ask for healing, if it is in God's sovereign will. It is a wonderful time for myself, and I was able to speak of the small group, which do not attend our church, and iron out those issues. If needed, my husband comes with me and receives prayer too!" – Kathy*

It should also be noted that each individual's medical choices should be respected. Taking medication does not mean that a person lacks faith. God is the great physician, but He also has equipped human physicians with knowledge and skills. Willie says, "I still take pain medications, and I was *chastised* by the church at one point for my lack of faith." This is unfortunate as well as incorrect behavior.

God Does Heal... Sometimes

God can and does heal people every day. Let us not forget this fact and praise Him for it.

> *"I had hypoglycemia and had been on a strict diet for over nine months. At a Bible study, one of the little old ladies had prepared cinnamon rolls. She was very upset that I couldn't eat them and said 'God can take of that' laid her little hands on me and prayed a simple prayer and I was surprised to find that I was indeed healed! It had not one thing to do with my faith, for sure! I guess maybe God liked the lady's cinnamon rolls! I suspect God really liked that little old lady, who is now with Him. Another time, I had been diagnosed with rheumatoid arthritis and was really suffering in my knees. I attended a healing mission at church and was surprised to be called out as one who had recently gotten that diagnosis. Only one person there knew I'd had that diagnosis and she was not a member of the church. Yes, I was healed and the evidence was I could kneel to pray which I had not been able to do in months. I believe there are lessons to be learned in some illness that I might not learn otherwise. I would like to be healed of chronic fatigue syndrome and to have energy, but until that happens, I pray that God helps me learn, and I lift up the pain and weakness for the salvation of others. Maybe my prayers at those times will help others in some way. In some ways, that helps relieve the guilt and loss that I feel, because a lot of the time my concentration is so bad that I cannot pray." – Virginia*

We Must Understand That the Lord Chooses to Heal in Different Ways, Not Just Physically

> *"I have pulled through more crises and troubles than I can tell. I think my biggest miracle of all was the emotional healing I received from the Lord. I was a Spirit-filled Christian and ministering full-time when I became seriously sick. I then went through a wilderness period that was most unbearable. After my 28th hospitalization I wanted to give up. Emotionally and spiritually I was dead. God healed me. I now know His grace. I now have peace and joy, depression is hardly ever a problem. I know more of His Word than ever. I have learned to keep my shield up from the condemnation attacks. I love to minister God's grace to chronically sick people. The emotional realm always needs healing and in this area I see dramatic results. I have witnessed miracles of healing – amazing things – and I know God heals. But for every one of those I see over a thousand who are not physically healed. I do know that emotional healing can be almost one-hundred percent when one ministers compassion and grace to the individual freeing them from condemnation. When a physically ill person is set free in their soul and spirit, they experience less pain physically. I know that as fact because I have experienced it." – Jenny*

Chapter 3

Tim Hansel writes in his book *You Gotta Keep Dancin'*
"I have prayed hundreds, if not thousands, of times for the Lord to heal me—and he finally healed me of the need to be healed. I had discovered a peace inside the pain. I finally came to the realization that if the Lord could use this body better the way it is, then that's the way it should be. I'm quite sure I would be a different person were it not for my accident."

"I have been to many healing services and have been prayed over many times. I believe that God has touched me in some way, but I have not received the physical healing that I personally would wish for. I also believe that suffering has a purpose and is not necessarily something to run from (although my human nature wants to), but rather something to embrace for Jesus' sake if it happens to exist. If a healing is to occur it must be for His glory, not just to make our lives easier. Maybe some of us suffer so that others can practice their Christian charity on us? It is difficult to accept this help many times, but then that helps us to grow in humility. I don't know the answer here, but would encourage anyone with chronic pain to be prayed over/with as often as the opportunity presents itself. We don't always see any visible results, as a matter of fact, most times we don't, but prayer is never wasted. Never cease to pray for healing, but realize that in the end it is God's will, not ours. In some way our suffering is a help to our souls, if not God would not allow it."
—Janine

"I have been prayed for many times and sought prayer for healing many times, and I think that is why I am not as afflicted as others with this disease. I believe that the Lord has used this disease to draw me closer to him, and for his purposes has kept me needy."
—Bonnie

"I see my pain as a blessing (although I wouldn't have chosen it) in relating to many people as I've been in my field of therapy. God teaches me ways to cope, real-life things I can do, and I in turn have been able to pass on these ideas as I've worked in chronic pain clinics for ten years and now am in private practice." —Ellie

"I love the Lord Jesus Christ with all of my heart and soul, and I know that He could heal me in a moment if he wanted to. He could provide the cures for diabetes, cancer, aids, lupus, or any other diseases if He so chose to do so. I also believe that he uses all things (good or bad) for his purposes, and for his glory. People just don't understand unless they too have experienced a disability."
—Donna

Healing is a complicated issue, and there are so many strong opinions regarding it. Entire books have been written on the subject, and even they seem somewhat incomplete. This is definitely an area where greater understanding is needed by all individuals.

"I believe churches need to teach on healing and what happens when it doesn't come. There are many controversial points on healing. I had a small group of people call me and want me to attend a healing school.

The idea is to 'speak the word' and constantly be running scripture through your head day and night, claiming God's word. The more seed (God's word) you receive in you, be prepared for more pain, because Satan attacks you then even more and You have to fight the battle. I just wasn't sure about this." —Kathy

---

1. Hurst, Jane. "Disability from the Point of View of Religion and Spirituality" in *Disability Studies Quarterly,* Summer 1995, Volume 15, No. 3.
2. Beibel, David. *How to Help a Heartbroken Friend*, 1996. New Spire Publishing.
3. Hurst, Jane. "Disability from the Point of View of Religion and Spirituality" in *Disability Studies Quarterly,* Summer 1995, Volume 15, No. 3.
4. Hansel, Tim. *You Gotta Keep Dancin'*. 1998. Chariot Family Publishing.

Chapter 3

Chapter 4
What Exactly is Chronic Illness/Pain Ministry?

<u>ESSENTIAL #4 Chronic Illness/Pain ministry is More Than Delivering Meals.</u>
In this chapter you will learn:
- *Chronic Illness/Pain ministry takes a change in awareness, attitude, and actions.*
- *The importance of having ministries that meet all kinds of needs: physical, relational, spiritual and emotional.*
- *Why people who live in pain want to participate in church and ministries, and how they can use their gifts.*

When you first picked up this book and started to read, you may have thought that chronic illness/pain ministry was as simple as getting a group of people together who were hurting and talking about the pain. As you read through chapter 3, however, you probably realized just how many issues there are when in comes to the spiritual community and living with chronic pain. And you may be thinking, "I never knew there were so many assumptions about illness, healing, and how to minister to someone with a chronic illness. How can I help? How can I make more people understand?"

Chronic illness/pain ministry is much more than gathering a group of people in a room and debating about why God has allowed them to have an illness. Chronic illness/pain ministry is more than someone in the church asking an ill person, "How are you feeling?" Chronic illness/pain ministry involves a change in awareness, attitude and actions. It involves knowing what people who live with illness would like from their church and establishing ministries to meet those needs.

The Invisibility of Chronic Illness

Living with an invisible chronic illness can mean constantly trying to redefine your condition. Those with illness can't keep up with the rest of the world, and yet the world sees no excuse for their lack of participation. Some would argue that having an *invisible* chronic illness could be a blessing, as one has a choice to tell others or remain an assumed normal person. The disadvantage of this is trying to convince others that the disease is legitimate and painful. Many people think "Aren't you overdoing it... or playing it up a bit?" People's observations do not conform to their expectations as to what a sick person should look and act like. Therefore, they are quick to become intolerant and suspect that the symptoms are overstated.

"Because my lung disease is invisible, people at church have said some unkind things like 'Get on with your life; go back to work full time if you expect to

eat. The bible says if you do not work you are not entitled to eat.' My specific lung diseases have constant pain involved with them due to the fibrosis. Lungs, however, are not visible so people assume you are faking it. It's been very difficult to deal with degenerating health and this as well. I almost stopped going to church entirely, but I know that God knows the truth and that this would be wrong." – Arles

It is often not only the disease itself that is painful, but the emotional effects of having the illness discounted, having one's respectability and judgement questioned, and dealing with the criticism of others. It is extremely necessary for the person with chronic illness to feel that their disease is validated, even by people who they don't know.

"At leadership meetings in the last couple of months, during our time of prayer or discussions prior to the prayer, I have heard things like, 'I believe that people are sick or have health problems because they have buried an anger deep inside of them and have become bitter about it' (something unresolved in their past). I have also heard, 'If you believe, you will be well or healed.' Or, 'Claim God's promises, and you will be healed.' These types of comments really hurt me. It is as though they are telling me that there must be something wrong with my relationship with the Lord, or that my faith is not strong enough if I do not receive a healing from God. I continue to work on my relationship with my Lord. It is an ongoing process for me. Why don't people accept persons with chronic illnesses? When remarks like those above are said, it makes me feel as though God cannot use me because I am flawed in some way. I feel as though I am not good enough to serve Him." – Donna

Most people in the church are well meaning, caring, concerned individuals. So why do they say such hurtful things? Most times, they just aren't aware of the fact that what they are saying is demeaning and harmful. People become awkward around people who are suffering and they don't know what to say. Instead of saying nothing, they try to help the ill person or fix the problem. Unfortunately, advice and hollow encouragement is often the last thing an ill person wants to hear. Usually they just want someone who is willing to listen.

"One of the most important things people could do as my friend, is to be more aware of what not to say, and just listen." – Cori

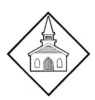

We Don't Feel Like How We Look

"Not all who 'look' healthy are healthy. From my looks you'd think I was never ill, unless you look into my dead eyes." – Virginia

"I have a handicap sticker on my car because I cannot walk far without arrhythmia's. Sometimes I get looks, because I am only 39 years old and I park where the elderly are at church. I get glares, as if I am taking a disabled person's spot! I have even been yelled at." – Jenny

"One feels awkward having to explain yourself all the time. Certain individuals in the church have made it blatantly clear that they do not believe I have a terminal illness, although I have had 54 hospitalizations in my life; 44 in the last six years." – Debra

One would believe that pain would be socially understood and somewhat sympathized with. Although people do sympathize with pain, it is under circumstances that we believe are severely painful, such as childbirth, trauma, late stages of cancer, etc. People cannot relate with the chronically ill since the individual is not screaming, crying or grimacing. We, who live with chronic pain, often walk, talk, and function normally (as far as can be seen) so it is assumed that the pain is overstated. Migraines, for example, are often misunderstood as being just a bad headache. For those who experience them, their whole world comes to a halt until the pain subsides. Fortunately, "The Lord does not look at the things man looks at. Man looks at the outward appearance, but the Lord looks at the heart" (I Samuel 16:7b).

David Beibel shares in his book *How to Help a Heartbroken Friend*, a story about a woman who faced tragedy in her life.

> "Friends and acquaintances literally walked away, crossed the street, turned around in a store aisle, quickly walked past me and so on. I expected they would be there for us and let us hurt. I know they care, but simply have no understanding of how to demonstrate that. Love is not enough; it has to be love with action. Love enough to carry a piece of my pain as they share my hurt. The church was our major social life, so our social structure fell apart. We were just plain ignored by most of our church, judged by some. I really struggle with the realization that my non-Christian friends have been much more *there* than my Christian friends. Why?"

There is no doubt that a need exists in our Christian community to change the way we react and respond to people who live with illness or pain. So, where do we start?

Ways That a Church Can be Educated About Invisible Chronic Illness:

- Have the pastor address illness related issues in sermons; include issues such as "When a person isn't healed…" as described in chapter 3.
- Have a present chronic illness ministry in the church that is *visible* and active.
- Have brochures available on the church resource table. For example, … And He Will Give You Rest has a brochure available called *"When a Friend Has a Chronic Illness: What to Say, How to Help."*
- Keep church leaders informed about people who have invisible chronic illnesses.

Before mentioning the ways in which you can assist a chronically ill person, it should be noted that **before doing anything,** the person should be **asked** if they would like help. There are a variety of people who will respond to help

in different ways:
- The person who has a great deal of pride and is hesitant to ask for, or even accept help, under any circumstances.
- The person who would love assistance, but will deny it. For example, if you just bring her dinner, she will graciously accept, but she would never have accepted it otherwise.
- The person who, when asked how she can be helped, will give you some specific or general ways that would be of assistance and give thank you for the offer.
- The person who has had her life turned upside down by her illness, feels totally out of control, and wants to be allowed to make all decision so that she can to still maintain some control in her household.
- The person who is tired of people making assumptions about what she wants and doesn't want. She'd just like to be consulted.

How do you accommodate all of these personalities? The best way is to volunteer to do something specific, and confirm that it is okay.

For example:

Don't ask: "Is there anything that I can do to help out?" *(She will l likely answer "no, thanks. I'm fine.")*

Do ask: "I noticed your lawn is getting about as tall as mine. I wouldn't mind coming over and cutting it for you Saturday afternoon. Would that be helpful for you?" *(She'll likely answer "yes" and be grateful for your offer.)*

Don't ask: "Let me know if you need me to run any errands for you this week."

Do ask: "I'm going to be going to the pharmacy and grocery store Tuesday afternoon. I'd be happy to pick up whatever you need. Just make a list of anything you can think of. Would that be helpful for you?"

Have Ministries that Serve Physical Needs

It probably comes as no surprise that we start with physical needs. James wrote, "What good is it, my brothers, if a man claims to have faith, but has no deeds? Suppose a brother or sister is without clothes and daily food. If one of you says to him, 'Go, I wish you well; keep warm and well fed,' but does nothing about his physical needs, what good is it? In the same way, faith by itself, if it not accompanied by action, is dead" James 2:14-17.

> *"When I had double pneumonia a number of years back, the church asked if they could prepare some meals. Well, I wasn't eating much of anything. My husband had stocked up on TV dinners and he was working a lot of overtime, so he wasn't home to eat much of what they would have prepared. We declined graciously, but with gratitude." – Ellie*

So now you know how to go about asking, but what can you do to help out?

> *"I would love to have someone offer to help with tasks and cleaning. I very often feel quite guilty that I cannot do these things. My husband gets overburdened, and quite frankly he doesn't care as much about order and uncluttered space as I do. So, this would be wonderful!"* – Cherie

> *"My house is no where near as clean as I would like and it's starting to get truly dirty in the corners. This really bothers me, but I can't find the energy for this on top of everything else. I have consciously made the decision to place this last on my list of priorities, but a cleaner house would do much in the way of giving me a sense of peace."* – Connie

It's true. For some reason women really do receive some peace from knowing that the corners of their home is clean. They feel like they are providing a home for their family. To someone who doesn't live with chronic illness, a clean house may seem like a strange request, but for women who have their abilities slowly diminishing, sometimes a house without cobwebs can make them feel like they are holding it all together. Having these feelings be acknowledged (by action) will truly minister to them.

Some housecleaning ministries are done anonymously. A group of women get the key from the husband or a neighbor and come in and clean quickly and leave. Some women enjoy not knowing who it was who saw the dust bunnies in the bedroom and the mildew around the tub.

Yardwork

There is no doubt that a chronically ill person rarely can mow his or her lawn or trim the branches. This may be an excellent project for a senior high or junior high youth group.

> *"I could use help with yard work in summer but no one even volunteers or asks if I need help, so I struggle on. The one time I did ask, I was told they had to spend their time with people who were really in need, not people who just thought they were in need. I never asked again."* – Anne   (oops! There's that invisible illness issue again!)

Babysitting

> *"For someone to take my extremely hyper 7-year-old whenever possible would be a help. Although I love her completely, she saps my energy faster than anything else and she could use the extra stimulation, company and attention that someone with more energy could give her sometimes."* – Bonnie

Babysitting, even for brief periods of time, is extremely helpful for people who live with illness. As stated above, people often don't have the energy to do everything with their children that they would like. They can rarely play ball, throw a Frisbee®, or walk through the zoo. Having someone occasionally spend some time with the child not only gives the parent a break, but also gives the child the opportunity to spend time with an energetic Christian adult. People in the church who have children should be aware of the parent's illness and invite the child to join them on outings or to their

Chapter 4

house to play for an afternoon. This small gesture can make a huge difference.

Errands

Running a few errands may not seem like much of a big deal, but sometimes they are the hardest things to coordinate. The best way to try to organize this is to have someone in charge of knowing what needs done on a weekly and monthly basis and then recruit volunteers to take these tasks on. Sometimes the ill person would like to get out, but driving is too difficult. If this is the case, it can be made into an event, such as getting your hair done together or having lunch while the oil in the car is being changed. If she is looking for information about her illness, volunteer to take her to the bookstore or library.

Have Ministries that Meet Relational Needs

"I think it would be great if they organized groups of Christians with chronic illness in support-type groups." – Cori

A small group or support group for people who live with chronic illness or pain is an excellent place to start. You may be surprised at the response you will get when you announce that a chronic illness/pain support group is forming. People will sign up who you never realized dealt with pain. There is an undeniable need in all of us to have the support of friends, and for those of us who live with chronic illness, the need to have people who understand what we are going through is even greater.

"My best experiences at church have been with my home study group, who remind me I'm not whining if I mention I'm hurting--even if it's every week! Also, those people who ask me how I really am." – Cheri

A support group offers a refuge where a person can come and honestly share what s/he is going through and know that others will nod in agreement, share their own experiences, and what they have learned.

"I depend on other people, when I have prolonged bouts of pain, to help me focus on other things. It helps me to remember that the pain isn't really all that important and that I can still have a semblance of a life. It does not have to be controlled by pain!" – Bonnie

Oftentimes those of us who live with chronic pain may already be "plugged in" at church, involved in a bible study, a worship team, or other ministry, but we rarely feel comfortable sharing our pain even in that group of fellow Christians. When we are living with our pain every day, we feel awkward asking for prayer every week. Yet at the same time, we desperately need prayer and emotional support.

"Almost on a daily basis I am in pain, although some days are better than others. The leadership group that I belong to have known about my physical problems since last April, but they do not seem sensitive to what I am going through. We have a time of prayer every Monday evening praying for those

who are sick, those having surgery or recovering from surgery, those with cancer, etc. For a while now, I have not mentioned any discomfort that I am experiencing, because I feel that they do not want to be bothered with it."
— *Donna*

Being around a group of Christians whom one can be totally honest with can make all of the difference in how one copes with the illness. Chronic illness is permanent and oftentimes degenerative, but if we have emotional/spiritual/relational support our journey will be much more rewarding.

"There are a few people at church who I know live with chronic illness. When I am around them it feels like I can truly be myself. When they say, 'How are you?' I can answer honestly instead of saying 'fine, thanks.' When they share with me that they are dreading their vacation because of all of the traveling involved, I understand. I don't shallowly say, 'You have nothing to worry about. You will have fun.' Instead I say, 'I'll pray for you,' and I really mean it. Nothing can replace this kind of relationship." — *Lisa*

Have Ministries that Meet Spiritual Needs

"Being on the prayer list always gives me more hope!" — *Cori*

People who live with chronic illness awake each day to pain, fatigue, new side effects from medications, visits to doctors, frustrations with the medical world, and loneliness. Even though they may be Christians and have a relationship with God, they have doubts, they wonder why God doesn't heal them, they get frustrated that people don't understand what they are going through, and they get mad at God. As we all do, they need spiritual growth, and when they are trapped in a body that doesn't want to function and sometimes trapped in a home, unable to get out, they are unable to be fed the Word of God and be reminded that God loves them and has not abandoned them.

Perhaps one or more of these ideas would work for your church.

"Encourage people, if they can, to host a small bible study group (run by someone else) in their home. That was very helpful for me because it gave me something to look forward to, motivated me to keep the house clean, let me sit in my comfortable chair, and I could drop into bed or the tub as soon as they left." — *Ellie*

"If they have a computer, share some of the helpful places on the net that you find of interest/encouragement. I've found the daily devotionals at Family Radio, Back to the Bible and Radio Bible Class to be something I look forward to reading. I'm sharing them with others now." — *Alice*

When a group of people who live with chronic illness were asked in what ways the church could minister to their spiritual needs they gave us a number of idea. These are shared on the following page.

Chapter 4

- Establish prayer partners for people with illness, within the church.
- Have a special visitation team that can keep in touch with people who live with chronic illness, to pray with them, see how they are doing, etc.
- Set up a buddy system so that at least one person from church calls them weekly to help them keep in touch.
- Establish a tape ministry to enable them to still hear the Word.
- Set up Bible studies in their homes with someone else preparing the coffee and teaching the lesson so that the ill person can still be part of it without any added stress being put on them.
- Organize a church library and a tape lending library and employ a volunteer to go around to the homes, perhaps once a month, to make material available to people who live with chronic illness.
- Ask the youth group to visits and bring their enthusiasm and music to people who live with chronic illness.

Have Ministries that Meet Emotional Needs

"My friends at church come to see me after the service and give me hugs. They are being really supportive and even call my place to see how I'm doing if I don't make it to church for a few weeks."
– Cori

In 2002, Rest Ministries began National Invisible Chronic Illness Awareness Week, as an annual week to educate others about invisible illness. Working together with other organization, Rest Ministries is the official sponsor, and as an organization we seek to outreach to people who are hurting and feeling as though no one understands what they are going through. This fourth week in September of each year is an excellent time to have the pastor do a sermon on chronic pain, have someone in the church share his testimony, or kick off a HopeKeepers group. See www. invisibleillness.com for more information.

What most people would like is fairly simple: They want know someone cares. They are reminded all too often that no one seems to understand what they are coping with, but if they knew someone cared, that could make a big difference in their state of mind and perspective on life.
A common quote today is "People don't care how much you know until they know how much you care."

"Postcards and offers of small favors would be wonderful. I hate the obvious stuff...'how are you?' questions, etc. because I usually can't answer 'fine' honestly so either I lie, or I say 'so-so' and then they want all of the details and I get all those 'poor you' looks. They are nice for sympathy sake, but make me feel like I am a whiner. Less asking and more little-tiny kindnesses, without all the explanation, needed would go a long way." – Amy

Here are a few ideas of ways to emotionally support someone in your church; some churches call this group of volunteers "HopeKeeper Helpers."
- Send notes or postcards periodically just to let her know someone is thinking of her.
- Have someone call her occasionally just to see how she is doing, but keep the conversations short.
- Have a children's Sunday school class send her a packet of pictures they have drawn for her.
- Have someone take her out to lunch occasionally.
- Have a few caring people <u>schedule</u> a visit, to bring Sunday's tape from church services. (Keep the visit short.)
- Invite people with chronic illnesses to speak at church group meetings to educate people on what frustrations, joys, trials and successes they have in spite of their illness.

Encourage Participation in Church and Ministries

"The church should realize that people with chronic illness/pain are a gift to the church in the same way that anyone else is. In many ways we, too, can minister, if allowed to within our own capabilities. For instance, many of us spend more time in prayer because we can't physically keep ourselves constantly busy. The church community could take advantage of that, maybe giving us special prayer intentions to lift up." – Connie

There are many ways that people in pain can be of service to the church. For their well being, it could be considered vital. Each person should be encouraged to find an area of ministry where he or she can become involved and enjoy. Having the opportunity to give to others will also make them feel more comfortable when they receive assistance from the church.

"Unlike acute illnesses, chronic illness don't often get better, but each person learns to adjust to their limitations over time. Often we are still able to function with limitations and the most important thing that the church can do is to respect those limitations, but allow us to still feel part of the body." – Lisa

One person said that a church leader told her, "When you first came to our church, it seemed you would be such an asset. And now you are one of those people who is always needing something." This attitude needs to be avoided at all costs. Each person is a gift from God and as Ephesians 2:10 says, "We are God's workmanship, created in Christ Jesus to do good works, which God prepared in advance for us to do." Those who live with illness are no exception.

"I would not want the focus from the church to be on my pain and illness, but rather I would like them to make use of the skills I have even with limitations. I would like to be informed of events at the church and be part of a prayer chain, and generally made to feel part of the congregation, whether I was there every Sunday or not." – Bonnie

Chapter 4

"My area of ministry is to send a personal note to someone who is having a difficult time, because I can relate to them and I feel for them. These are the ones I lean towards praying for because, again, I can relate." – Ellie

"I have found that the best thing that has helped me is when I receive the necessary help that I need to make it through the day. I have three children and am disabled. I want so much to be as normal and independent as possible, but that requires a lot of help. Right now, I have a group of ladies that come weekly to help me with housework. Once, when I was bedridden for a year, I had a family assigned to our family every night of the week for the final three months until I became more stable. They brought meals, babysat, played with my children, cleaned, and took a lot of the stressload off of our family. All illness responds to stress and improves when conditions are less stressful. In the emotional realm I have discovered that the best help for me was to see that I was still a person of value. Even in my weak condition I have an important role in the body of Christ. Although I may not be able to sing or help on physical projects, I was able to encourage, teach, pray and let His love shine through me in other ways. It feels good to feel needed by someone else and not just a burden. The enemy attack that I struggle with would be condemnation, and it is so wonderful for people to show compassion rather than being treated as an outcast or someone to be pitied. I thrive on encouragement just like a healthy person does." – Jenny

---

1. Beibel, David. *How to Help a Heartbroken Friend*, 1996. New Spire Publishing. (pg. 57).

Chronic Illness/Pain Ministry Plan for

_____
(your church)

Chronic illness/pain ministry coordinator _____

Physical coordinator _____

Duties: Find out what needs exist, recruit volunteers and coordinate assistance.

Relational coordinator_____

Duties: Organizem and facilitate "HopeKeepers" small group and coordinate with volunteers.

Spiritual coordinator _____

Duties: Determine ways to encourage spiritual growth and support and organize such ministries.

Emotional needs coordinator _____

Duties: Determine ways to emotionally support people who live with illness/pain and organize such ministries.

Participation coordinator _____

Duties: Determine ways to encourage people who live with illness or pain to participate in the church and organize such ministries.

Chronic Illness/Pain Outreach Ministry Sign-Up

Name _____

Address _____

Phone number _____

I would be able to contribute in the following ways: *(please check)*

Number of hours per week I can volunteer my time. _____

- ☐ Running errands
- ☐ Making a meal
- ☐ Visiting someone in their home
- ☐ Babysitting
- ☐ Making a telephone call
- ☐ Being an emergency contact
- ☐ Yard work
- ☐ Repairs
- ☐ House cleaning
- ☐ Sending encouraging notes.
- ☐ Administrative (helping organize other volunteers)

Thank you! Someone will be contacting you.

Chronic Illness/Pain Outreach Ministry Sign-Up

Name _____

Address _____

Phone number _____

I would be able to contribute in the following ways: *(please check)*

Number of hours per week I can volunteer my time. _____

- ☐ Running errands
- ☐ Making a meal
- ☐ Visiting someone in their home
- ☐ Babysitting
- ☐ Making a telephone call
- ☐ Being an emergency contact
- ☐ Yard work
- ☐ Repairs
- ☐ House cleaning
- ☐ Sending encouraging notes.
- ☐ Administrative (helping organize other volunteers)

Thank you! Someone will be contacting you.

Sample Article for Your Church Newsletter

When someone in our church has surgery, most of us quickly respond. We deliver flowers, we make hospital visits, and send get-well cards. Oftentimes a prayer chain is started and meals and childcare is provided. We all rejoice when the person recovers and returns to his or her normal life. Nearly 100 million people in the U.S., however, have a physical *chronic condition*. Two-thirds of adults ages 45 to 65 and one-third of adults ages 18-44 live with a chronic disease; Contrary to popular perceptions, the elderly represent less than one-third of those who have chronic conditions that cause limitations and disabilities.

With this in mind, *(your church)* will be establishing a chronic illness/pain ministry. *(Name of coordinator)* will be coordinating this ministry and is looking forward to hearing from those of you who live with chronic conditions or pain. Over the next *(few months)* we will be listening to what you would like to see in this new ministry. We are also actively seeking volunteers to assist. Whether you can spend two hours a month running errands or writing a few encouraging postcards, we need you!

If you have a chronic condition or would like to volunteer please contact *(Name of coordinator)* at *(coordinator's phone number)* or sign up on *(date)* at *(location)*.

Here are some encouraging statistics:
- Looking at a variety of illnesses from cardiovascular conditions to cancer, researchers found that frequent attendance at worship services was linked to healthier lives.
- Up to 80 percent of all patients feel they have a spiritual dimension to their lives that they would like to be taken into account by their doctors.
- 95% of physicians said they had treated patients who believed that religious activities improved their physical condition
    (The National Institute for Healthcare Research.)

Permission to reprint.
"Sample article for your church newsletter"
So You Want to Start a Chronic Illness/Pain Ministry ©1997

Chapter 5
The Etiquette of Chronic Illness: Knowing What to Say and Not to Say

ESSENTIAL #5: *Knowing What to Say and Not Say Can Make a Difference*
In this chapter you will learn:
- *How to know what not say to a person in pain and why it's important.*
- *How to teach people in your church about illness etiquette.*
- *What to say and what you can do to help a person in pain.*

> *"My reason for going back to church after many years away was to find supportive people who I thought would be understanding. After choir rehearsals, we always ask for prayer requests. Often there is a death in a family, or someone has just been diagnosed with cancer or the like, but there is never any mention of those of us who suffer quietly every day. I have asked for help to endure the constant pain I am in. There has only been one woman (who also has lupus) who has ever asked me how I was feeling or if she could help in any way. Most just see my 'apparent' healthy smile and assume I am perfectly well. I don't expect people to fuss over me or make a big issue; I just wish for someone to talk to when I have really bad days or when the requirements of singing in the choir are absolutely everything I can muster for one service. (Like climbing 2 flights of stairs.) I had hoped Christian people would be more sensitive to the needs of people in pain. Maybe if there was more information and ways of letting concerned people know how to help, people like myself could be more open and discuss things with others."* – Lynette

If you don't have a chronic condition, you may be wondering why this chapter is necessary. After all, aren't people being a little too sensitive if it takes a whole chapter to inform others about how to act around them?

Well...yes and no. Granted, there will be times when we all stick our foot in our mouth and say something that doesn't come out the way we had planned. Other times, we are just ignorant, and we don't realize that we are saying something that could be hurtful. There are also the moments when we know that we may be crossing the line, but we are tired of "sick people always being so needy; somebody needs to tell them to get over it and quit looking for free help." We all have moments of sinful attitudes, and even if you live with chronic illness yourself, you've likely felt tired of illness and all that it entails being such a daily regime.

According to Rev. Dale Robbins, studies have shown that a great percentage of persons who cease attending church do so because of some type of offense or injury to their feelings that happened in church. Robbins says, "Some of these occur because of the insensitivity of the church; other times, people are at fault for being too touchy or sensitive to misunderstandings."

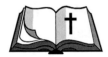

We must remember that we are made in the image of Christ. Philippians 2:2-4 says, "Then make my joy complete by being like-minded, having the same love, being one in spirit and purpose. Do nothing out of selfish ambition or vain conceit, but in humility consider others better than yourselves. Each of you should look not only to your own interests, but also to the interests of others."

It's important to be aware of what others are going through and their interests, because we are their siblings in Christ. Knowing how to make a person feel loved and cared for should be at the top of our priority list.

"Be wise in the way that you act toward outsiders; make the most of every opportunity. Let your conversation be always full of grace, seasoned with salt, so that you may *know how to answer everyone*" (Colossians 4:4-6). It is vital that when we speak to both Christians and non-Christians we represent our Savior in a way with which He would be pleased.

It's also important that we be careful to not give our opinion about things that we know little or nothing about. Philip Yancey, author of *Where is God When it Hurts?* writes, "Perhaps the most unsettling aspect of the book [of Job] is that the arguments of Job's friend sound suspiciously like those offered by Christians today....God dismissed all of Jobs' friends' high-sounding theories with a scowl. 'I am angry with you and your two friends, God said to one, 'because you have not spoken of me what is right, as my servant Job has" (Job 42:7) (1).

How do I Know What to Say or Not to Say?

In order to know the "secret language" of what to say and what not to say, one must have a chronic illness himself or live with a person who has a chronic illness. If you are reading this book in order to start a chronic illness/pain ministry at your church, and you do not have a chronic condition, it is vital that someone who does live with pain or illness volunteers to co-coordinate with you. Why is this so important?

True empathy cannot be learned out of a book or manual. No matter how many books you read about illness or how many support group meetings you attend, if you do not have it, you cannot understand the emotions involved. When it comes to spiritual guidance, there are personal feelings that a leader must be in tune with in order to have an effective ministry.

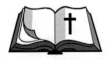

What Not to Say
Avoid giving "spiritual happy pills." Avoid giving anything that resembles a "spiritual happy pill" as described by David Biebel in *If God is So Good Why Do I Hurt So Bad* (2). People often believe that your suffering is a direct result of a

Chapter 5

"spiritual problem" that you are experiencing; They believe that once you fix this problem by praying more, confessing your sins, repenting, going to church, reading the Bible, etc., you will be healed. This isn't a new attitude. Even Jesus' disciples asked Him "Who sinned, this man or his parents, that he was born blind?" [Jesus answers "Neither this man nor his parents sinned, but this happened so that the work of God might be displayed in his life" (John 8:2,3)]. If even the disciples were unable to comprehend that God rarely uses illness as punishment, is it any surprise that people today still believe this?

Here are some examples of "spiritual happy pills":

"Spiritual Happy Pills"	*What an ill person thinks*
"Poor health is a sign of sin. You must have some kind of hidden sin in your life."	You're obviously blaming me for my illness. I can't cope with people who do that. I don't know if I will return to this church.
"If you would just confess your sins to God, I'm sure he would heal you."	I have confessed all that I know to confess. What happened to God's grace?
"You're obviously not spending enough time in the Word. Haven't you read, 'Ask and you will receive'? You need to claim it!"	I *have* asked for God's healing, and He has not given it to me. I'm also reading the Word. Maybe you don't remember how Paul asked three times for his thorn to be removed and God said, "My grace is sufficient."
"You must not be praying for healing right. Either you don't have enough faith or you aren't asking for the right thing. Have you used the oil like it says in James?"	She thinks that God can only heal me by using the oil? Maybe I don't have enough faith. Where am I going wrong, Lord? Something must be wrong with me if you aren't answering my prayers.
"All sickness is evil. It's never from God. God never wants us to suffer."	I'm doing the best I can. How can this evil have so much control over my life when I am trying so hard to do as God desires?

Avoid Giving "God balm."

Although people are trying to say encouraging things in this awkward situation, they often forget that the person in pain is experiencing real

Chapter 5

emotional turmoil and doesn't want to hear blanket statements that seem to avoid the emotions that he is feeling.

Below are some examples of "God balm."

"God balm"	What an ill person thinks
"Everything works together for good."	That's easy for you to say. You aren't the one that has to live with this. I know Romans 8:28 and I'd rather not have it quoted to me.
"I know that this isn't God's will for you."	How do *you* know what God's will is for me? No one really knows.
"Why would God let this happen to a nice person like you?"	I'm trying to figure that our myself. You must think that there is some reason I deserve it that you don't know about.
"God has chosen you to suffer for Him. You should be thanking Him for allowing you to bring glory to Him in this way."	Thanking Him? Some spiritual giants may be up to this, but right now I just want my old life back. This isn't how I had planned on serving God.
"I just know that you will be healed."	What if I'm not? I'm getting worse all of the time. Will she blame me if I'm not healed? She just doesn't have a clue!
"If you pray for God to heal you, I know he will answer your prayers."	I have been praying for healing and he's not answering my prayers. Maybe I'm not praying right. Maybe I don't have enough faith or something.
"There are so many people praying for you. God is going to answer our prayers in no time!"	What if he doesn't? How does she know that God will heal me? How will she treat me if her prayers aren't answered?

Can you think of some examples of God Balm? What have people said to you that felt like a "token response" despite their good intentions? Most of us have heard some of these. How have you responded?

Avoid Sharing Cures

Many people are tempted to share any and all information they hear on the news about any given illness. People who live with chronic illness are bombarded with news about vitamins, herbs, teas, pills, and alternative therapies. Church should be one place where they can be free from encountering this.

Those who live with chronic illness are generally well informed about their illness. They often have considered alternative treatments and are also consulting with their physicians regarding their treatment. They understand that the news shows broadcast anything they can get their hands on regarding new treatments or study findings, so they may seem hesitant to get excited about what they hear. They know that the study findings they hear about on the news or read about in the magazines are usually based on preliminary studies and that drugs or treatments are years away from FDA approval and distribution. They have learned how to live with their illness and take one day at a time.

> *"A woman at church cornered me after one service and told me she was really into health and had read a lot of books. One book had a chapter on arthritis that stated oftentimes arthritis was caused by food allergies. I tried to politely say, 'thanks for the information' and leave, but she kept trying to convince me I needed to change my diet. I finally held my deformed hand up in front of her face and said, 'Look! This is not a food allergy!' I didn't know what else to do to get her to stop harassing me."* – Lisa

If someone wants to share some information about treatment, this is the appropriate way to go about it:

If you must share something, mail the information to the person with a nice note, and never mention it again.

This can be hard to do because there is a little part in all of us that wants the recognition of being helpful. If you really care, however, know that even by mailing it you may cause offense, so be sure it's worth the risk of the relationship itself.

Why is it so Important to Avoid Saying the Wrong Thing?

When you are ministering to people who live with chronic illness, they are often dealing with depression, anger, fear and a multitude of other emotions. Each individual is on his or her own journey. The life of a person is severely impacted when she is diagnosed with a chronic illness, and her roles, dreams, attitudes, and emotions easily go spinning out of control. Getting out of bed,

Chapter 5

getting dressed and coming to church may be the biggest accomplishment she has made all week, and the last thing you want to do is to say something accusing, judgmental, ignorant, or hurtful.

These are some other things to be aware of:

What not to do:	*The comment made:*	*What an ill person thinks:*
Assume the illness is all a matter of attitude.	"When are you going to get rid of that wheelchair?"	Like I have any control over it? I don't want to be using a wheelchair!
Blame the person for the illness.	"Did you know that cancer is caused by stress?"	I didn't have *that* much stress, and I dealt with it just fine! Mind over body only goes so far!
Tell a person what she should and shouldn't feel.	"You shouldn't feel that way! That's ridiculous!"	See if I ever share my emotions with you again!
Pity a person.	"You poor thing. I just feel so sorry for you."	I don't want anyone's pity. I don't need those kinds of friends.
Share all of your sob stories to try to make the person feel grateful for her circumstances.	"I know exactly how you feel..." followed by a long discourse of your problems.	Here we go again... She has no idea how I feel! I think I will just tune out.
Avoid giving the person the opportunity to share her feelings and her fears.	"Let's talk about happier things. Let me read you a poem I brought."	"I really need to talk to someone who will just listen. Poems aren't going to make me feel any better."

Yancey writes in his book, *Where is God When it Hurts?*,
"I have interviewed many Christians with life-threatening illnesses, and every ones without exception, has told me how damaging it can be to have a visitor plant the thought 'You must have done something to deserve this punishment.' At the very moment when they most need hope and strength to battle the illness, they get instead a frosty dose of guilt and self-doubt. I'm glad the author of Job took such care to record the rambling conversations of Job's friends: that book serves as a permanent reminder to me that I have no right to stand beside a suffering person and pronounce, 'This is the will of God,' no matter how I cloak that sentiment in pious phrases" (3).

Chapter 5

Consequences of Saying the Wrong Thing

There are three likely consequences when a well-meaning individual says the wrong thing.

(1) The person will turn away from the individual who made the comment with anger, frustration, resentment and other negative feelings. If he is at all stumbling in his walk with God, he could easily refrain from attending church in the future, assuming that all Christians feel the same way.

> *"I have been approached by a number of well-meaning Christians in my church who have ignorantly made inconsiderate and inappropriate comments. These comments hurt to the core of my being. I struggle to let the conversation go and I pray that God will allow me to not take it personally, but it still hurts, and I find myself believing that 'no one understands!'"*
> *– Amy*

Although the comment is often made by an individual, one person can easily be seen as a representative of the entire church, and it can easily affect the future attendance of the ill person.

(2) The person in pain may believe the comments that an individual makes. "When you're in pain, the problem is that it is much easier to surrender to the accusers than to resist their assault," writes Biebel. "For one thing, you don't have the energy to resist. For another, you, like them, long for resolution."

As we struggle with our pain and the reasons behind it, it can become easier to grab onto self-condemnation than to have no answers at all. Dealing with the guilt that we have somehow brought it upon ourselves can actually be *easier* to cope with than the anxiety of not having any answers.

(3) On a rare occasion, comments may not affect a person at all. They may become numb to people's ignorance. This is, however, a very rare occurrence. No matter how often we hear insensitivity, we rarely become used to it.

> *"Those who have labored with me during these times are sympathetic mostly when I 'appear the part.' The rest of the time, although I am in constant pain trying not to complain, people avoid me when I am just going to talk about my illness. In order to have friends and fellowship, I have had to learn to pretend I am okay, which complicates things too."* *– Jenny*

There is no indication in scripture that a person with an illness or disability is loved any less than the rest of humankind, and therefore, they are as worthy of God's love as anyone else. The comments that people make are often out of fear, tradition, or peculiar interpretations of scripture that have been taken out of context. The mystery of human suffering and lack of fairness bewilders us all, and so often we are susceptible to making thoughtless statements that can be hurtful and accusing. Says Blair and Blair, "Oftentimes, the same well-intentioned religious professionals who walk roughshod over scripture and feelings of their congregants with disabilities are ignorant of their denomination's resources for help in these regards" (4).

So... What Can I Say?

It's obvious that people who are in physical pain or who have recently been diagnosed with a chronic condition need our support. Isn't that what you are reading this booklet for? So how do we help? One of the things that people need most is to be able to talk to someone who will just listen. They need someone who will give them a (gentle) hug. They need someone who will miss them when they are not there.

> *"I was in the first year of chronic fatigue syndrome and beginning to struggle even to attend church. I began feeling, with an unfriendly group around me, why bother to attend? The church was pretty dry anyway. So I just stopped going. Only one person called to see how we were doing. I've not attended services in almost ten years and there has been no contact with members who I thought were friends. I'd been a regular there for twelve years at the time I left. (This is a fairly small town.) Except now that I've found a new church home I seem to run into several of those old members who now tell me they miss me and are mad at me for changing churches."* — Bonnie

Author and lecturer Leo Buscaglia once talked about a contest he was asked to judge. The purpose of the contest was to find the most caring child. The winner was a four-year-old child whose next door neighbor was an elderly gentleman who had recently lost his wife. Upon seeing the man cry, the little boy went into the old gentleman's yard, climbed onto his lap, and just sat there. When his mother asked him what he had said to the neighbor, the little boy said, "Nothing, I just helped him cry." Perhaps what people in pain most need is a friend so close that they don't hesitate to cry with them.

> *"They need to feel God's love in the practical helps. Then they need to hear about grace. They need someone to listen to their plight and accept them in grace without running the opposite way to avoid them. They need to be needed in the church and have a part...for they are members and have a unique gift."* — Jenny

How to Help

- If you don't know what to say, just tell her that. Say "I wish I knew the right thing to say, but just know that I care, and I am here if you need me."
- Focus on her needs and not on your own discomfort of not having adequate answers.
- Be physically near her, and if it is appropriate, touch her hand or give her a hug.
- Keep your words brief.

- Let her express what she is feeling.
- Don't pretend that you don't have struggles.
- Assure her that you are praying for her.
- Ask her what she would like you to pray for.
- Encourage her to recall the times she has experienced God's faithfulness.
- Encourage her to take one day at a time.
- Encourage her to reach out for the help they need (friends, family, pastor).
- Help her to realize that coping with troubles takes time.
- Remind her of God's shepherding love (Ps. 23).
- Remind her of God's control over the universe, both the big and small events of life.
- Don't ignore her problem.
- Don't be artificial in trying to "cheer her up." Be genuine. Be the friend you were to them before trouble hit.
- Show her the love you would like other people to show you if you were in their situation. Be a good listener.
- Acknowledge how much she hurts.
- Give her time to heal. Don't rush the process.
- Send notes just to say you are thinking of her.

> *"When I became ill with myasthenia gravis, everyone found out. We had just moved to this small town of a thousand people, but word traveled fast. I started to get cards and notes from people. The one message in every one of them was that they were praying for me and my family. These are people that I may never have met or may have been introduced to only once. To know that so many people cared enough to take the time to send a card to let me know that they were praying for us made me feel so strong. No matter how bad I was feeling physically, I knew that my girls and my husband would have a town to care for them. I could concentrate on myself. This has strengthened my belief in the power of prayer."* – Sherrie

Have Realistic Expectations About What a Person Can Handle

People who live with invisible chronic illness are often expected to participate in or take responsibility for tasks, which they may not be able to do.

> *"I was a member of a very large Pentecostal church from the time I first developed problems with chronic illness and for almost ten years afterwards. I was in women's ministries, taught Wee College, led Bible studies and was co-leader of a ministry to people in economical and spiritual need. I was very involved in the church and very busy. As my disease progressed, my ability to maintain the busy schedule became less and less, and unfortunately, I found very little understanding from people at the church who's expectations were that I would always be able to fill the jobs I had initially chosen. As time went on, I could no longer physically maintain the hectic schedule. I had to spend time in the hospital, so I could not fulfill the obligations I had to these groups. I was made to feel that somehow I was responsible for leaving them short-*

Chapter 5

> *handed. When I was unable to go to church, sometimes for weeks at a time, I was basically abandoned by the friends I had there."* – Bonnie

Although no one can be expected to know every physical limitation of the people in the church, one can delegate by asking for volunteers, rather than assigning tasks. When a person signs up for a particular task, one shouldn't try to tell her that she needs to be doing something that is more physically demanding.

> *"I have been embarrassed because I have been asked to help get chairs or run errands. I am not physically able to. Someone with a visible broken foot that will heal in 8 weeks, however, gets a lot of loving attention: doors opened, help with carrying books, etc."* – Jenny

Most people don't expect friends to be lining up at their doorstep with meals and mowing their lawn for them every week. A friend recently shared, "I just needed to have someone be strong for me, since I couldn't be strong any more. I just wanted someone to sit beside me while I cried." This may feel awkward. People feel helpless. They think "There must be something more that I should be doing." There isn't. More than anything, people want to know someone cares.

> *"...Being aware and showing it in various ways, but not constantly asking how we are or if we are feeling better, because chances are, we are lousy and not feeling any better, and it is hard to always admit that. That is where education comes in. Asking what kind of week we are having and if there is anything they could do to help (make a casserole, take a kid for a couple hours, come do your vacuuming or cleaning baseboards or windows or one of those things that is very energy draining) would be much better."* – Connie

Chapter 6
Small Group Ministry: A Brief Overview

ESSENTIAL #6: You Must Have the
Right Motivations for Leading a Chronic Illness-Pain Ministry
In this chapter you will learn:
➤ Five characteristics of effective Bible discussion leaders
➤ If you're being called to small group leadership.
➤ The right and wrong motivations for being a small group leader.

> *"Being able to express myself without being afraid of judgement, because others with chronic illness would better understand where I am coming from, would be all the motivation I would need to join a group." – Bonnie*

> *"Managing a 'trip out' with as little consequences as possible is my daily goal. But it would be worth the extra suffering to be able to share with others like myself." – Lynette*

All of us need relationships. People who live with daily physical pain are likely to feel isolated, even when surrounded by loved ones. "No one knows what I am going through. No one understands!" is often said in frustration. Fortunately, a small group ministry can help take these feelings of loneliness and isolation away, as people are given the opportunity to socialize and grow with other Christians who also face the "thorn of illness."

"God didn't create us to be involved in a solo sport," Pastor Robenson says. "Christianity is a team sport. Personal involvement with other believers fosters spiritual growth by providing an environment of intimacy, encouragement and accountability."

Rest Ministries, Inc. is a ministry for people who live with chronic illness or pain and it has small groups throughout the United States called **HopeKeepers** (TM). **HopeKeepers** is a place where a person can feel safe. It's a sanctuary; a place where one can pour out their souls regarding everything in his or her life, but especially about the physical ailments.

Oftentimes when a person has an illness and is involved in a small group, surrounded by healthy individuals, the ill person may still feel like he is burdening the others with constant prayer requests about his physical condition. The group of people may kindly listen, but they still can't grasp what the ill person is going through, the challenges he or she faces, and the many choices that must be made. In a **HopeKeepers** small group, one can openly express these feelings and the group can gather around each individual and say, "We understand," and truly mean it.

Five characteristics of effective Bible discussion leaders

(1) *The characteristic of obedience.*
If you are considering becoming a leader or a small group, there are three things, which you must be right in relationship to. These are: (1) God, (2) God's Word, and (3) God's people and persons in position to authority.

(2) *The characteristic of prayer.*
People are looking for someone to pray for them and with them. Prayer is a vital part of our relationship with God.

(3) *The characteristic of belief.*
We need to have a faith that is enthusiastic. Without faith, we are unable to please God and therefore are of no direct benefit to others.

(4) *The characteristic of compassion combined with clear communication.*
Scripture tells us to speak the truth in love (Ephesians 4:15).

(5) *The characteristic of study and preparation.*
2 Timothy explains how leaders must be teachable in order to correctly handle the word of truth.

Are You Being Called to Small Group Leadership?

Do you have a growing and maturing relationship with the Lord? (See John 15:5)	❐ Yes	❐ No
Do you have a sense of calling from the Lord to serve people? (See John 21:15-17)	❐ Yes	❐ No
Do you have a vision for building up future leaders? (See 2 Timothy 2:2)	❐ Yes	❐ No
Do you want to glorify the Lord with whatever you do? (See Col. 3:23)	❐ Yes	❐ No
Do you want to bear fruit in your life? (See John 15:8)	❐ Yes	❐ No
Do you want to shepherd others and be an example? (See 1 Peter 5:2)	❐ Yes	❐ No

> *The most outstanding leaders are those with a compassionate touch. Their ministry is based on caring, not knowledge.*

Chapter 6

The Right and Wrong Motivations for Leading a Small Group

If you are considering leading a small group, take a moment to look at the reasons why. Did you answer yes to all of the questions on above? If so, you can be assured that you probably have the right motives for wanting to participate in small group leadership. If you answered no to some of them, you should examine your motives a little closer.

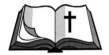

Do you want to lead a small group:
- **For self-exaltation?** The Bible says, "Let another praise you, and not yourself," (Proverbs 27:2).
- **To feel important or for the prestige?** We are not here to please man, but to please God. Look at your reasons for wanting prestige (1 Thess. 2:4-6).
- **Because someone has pressured you to do it?** Don't get involved with something that you don't have a passion for, because you won't last and you will not be an effective leader. 1 Peter 5:2 says "Be shepherds of God's flock that is under your care, serving as overseers, not because you must, but because you are willing, as God wants you to be."

Small groups are a wonderful place to build friendships with people that will last years. To lead a small group, you should be faithful, available and teachable. Don't worry about not being able to quote dozens of scriptures or having to go to the Bible to look up the answer to a question you encounter. As long as you are willing to look for the answers from the Bible and from church leadership, you are qualified to lead a small group. Talk to your the leaders in your church for more information about small groups.

Chapter 6

Notes

Chapter 7
How do I Answer Their Questions About "why?"

ESSENTIAL #7: You Don't Have to Have all the Answers
In this chapter you will learn:
- *No one has all of the answers.*
- *How to prepare for the questions you may receive.*

Before my first radio interview about *Rest Ministries*, I sat at my computer with a headset and four pages of notes. I was to be broadcast 3000 miles away in Florida and I was trying not to be nervous. I knew what I was going to talk about and I could recite my verses, stories and statistics without notes. If the interviewer asked me why I believed I had not been healed, I could easily answer that God had shown me a path in which I could reach out to other people who were hurting and bring glory to Him.

The interview went fine, and then the host said, "Let's take a few calls." What!? I wasn't prepared for this! Oh, please, God, don't let anyone get through that is going to ask me why God hasn't healed them. I tried to prepare for this, just in case, but I couldn't find the answer. How could I tell someone "God may be glorified more through your illness than your health?" How cold! That wasn't the way to make friends. Who was I to claim I knew what God's will is for an individual? Thankfully, there was only time for a Christian doctor to request information and no more calls made it through.

> *"Perhaps even more profound may be the conclusion that your faith will be stronger if you can't understand than if you do."*
> -David Biebel
> *If God is So Good, Why Do I Hurt So Bad?*

You are probably feeling the same way. "Who, me?! I don't know all of those verses about healing and I don't understand God's reasoning for suffering and pain. I could never help other people!" Those feelings that you are having are normal and, to be honest, I doubt I will ever find someone who truly can explain all the "whys" to me, because humans and God cannot be compared. Isaiah 55:8,9 says "Your thought are not my thoughts." Doesn't it stand to reason that God's logical

Chapter 7

explanation is not our logical explanation? Still, we must take a closer look and prepare, because just as the suffering will come, so too will the questions. This way, when we are encountered with them, we won't be surprised.

Unfortunately, none of these "answers" truly reveal the reasons a person is going through a difficult time. People may come to you and ask "Why is God doing this to me?" and I do not recommend that you hand them this booklet and say, "Here. The reason must be in this list somewhere." That would be cold, uncaring and you would be disappointed when you found out that not every "why" has a specific answer. The next two pages are a breakdown of some of the things that we do know about God and about suffering.

Use this as your guide when you encounter the "whys." Use it as a place to begin your understanding of God and suffering issues, but be aware that God doesn't reveal His purposes for every situation we will experience. David Beibel writes "Modern Christians sometimes rush to put His truth into little boxes, neatly systematized, categorized, and organized, and principalized, when God's perspective on suffering is too big for any of that. While for some, 'spirituality' is defined by what you know, for God it may be more how you handle what you *cannot* know."(1)

If God is All Powerful, Why Does He Let Bad Things Happen?

Some people may argue that the fact that there are good people who suffer proves that God is either not all-powerful or not all-good. Either way, they believe the Bible contradicts itself by claiming that God is both good and powerful. When we witness tragedy and unfairness we have the choice to either (1) deny that God is a personal God, concerned with our circumstances; (2) believe that God is good, but some things are beyond His control (as concluded by Rabbi Kishner in *Why Bad Things Happen To Good People)*; (3) believe that "whatever will be will be!" It must be God's will.

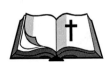

Here are some scriptures for you to read to better understand the character of God:
- God is pleased with those who do good, and slowly angers with those who resist Him. (Psalm 7:11; Nah. 1:1-7).
- God feels grief toward those who reject Him (Genesis 6:6; Psalm 95:10).
- God hurts when He must correct and punish us for our own good (Isaiah 63:9).
- God finds no pleasure in judging the wicked, and He hopes they will change their heart (Ezek. 18:23,32; 33:11).
- God finds delight in kindness, justice, and righteousness (Jeremiah 9:24).
- God loved the world so much that he became a part of humanity, in the form of Jesus Christ, and died like a sinner so that we could be saved (John 3:16; 2 Corinthians 5:21).

Chapter 7

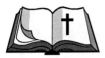

What Does God Control and What Does He Allow?

Here are some things we *do* know:
- **God is in control of history.** Paul declared that "He has made from one blood every nation of men to dwell on all the face of the earth, and has determined their preappointed times and the boundaries of their dwellings," (Acts 17:26).
- **God is active in history even when it seems He is not.** For example, more than 30 years after being the victim of his brothers' hatred, Joseph told them "Do not be afraid, for am I in the place of God. But as for you, you meant evil against me; but God meant it for good, in order to bring it about as it is this day, to save many people alive," (Gen. 50:19-20).
- **One may not easily be able to tell which part of history was God's doing and which was not since His actions are so interwoven with earthly and human factors.** We do know that he is a holy God who hates sin, therefore, He is never responsible for leading anyone to do evil. He can, however, work through our own human sin to accomplish His purposes.

Why Does God Allow Sickness and Disease?

We recognize that suffering can help us grow spiritually, (Hebrews 12:6) and yet some of the afflictions in life seem cruel and useless. If a baby is born with a deformity, who benefits? When a giving, caring, loving person is diagnosed with an illness, it doesn't seem fair. Oftentimes, it is hard for us to see the purpose behind the suffering that we encounter. Here are some main points to keep in mind.

"Always be prepared to give an answer to everyone who asks you to give the reason for the hope that you have."
1 Peter 3:15

- **There is a reason for each affliction, even though we cannot see it.** Jesus said that a man was born blind "that the works of God should be revealed in him," (John 9:3). Then Jesus healed the man. Up until this point, no one knew why the man had been blind, but God did. That was all that mattered. Sometimes, we must rest in the assurance that God knows the answer to the "why?" even when we do not. David Biebel writes in his book *If God Is So Good, Why Do I Hurt So Bad?*, "Perhaps even more profound may be the conclusion that your faith will be stronger if you *can't* understand than if you *do*."

- **We were never promised a perfect life here on earth.** Peter tells us in 1 Peter 4:12, "Dear friends, do not be surprised at the painful trial you are suffering, as though something strange were happening to you." Suffering is a direct result of sin's entrance into the world. Oftentimes, our troubles may be the side-effects of the sin that has entered our world, even though it is no fault of our own. In the New Testament, the apostle Paul described the whole creation of God as groaning and eagerly anticipating the time when it will be freed from the curse of decay and be remade, free from the effects of sin (Rom. 8:19-22).

Chapter 7

- **Suffering can be caused by other people.** Since God made us able to make free choices, we have made and will continue to make poor choices. When these choices are made they affect other people.

- **Suffering may be a product of Satan.** Job's life story is a vivid example of how a good person can suffer incredible tragedy because of satanic attack. God allowed Satan to take away Job's possessions, his family, and his health (Job 1,2). Job was a living testimonial to the trustworthiness of God. He illustrated that a person can trust God and maintain integrity even when one's life falls apart, because God is worth trusting. In the end, Job learned that even though he didn't understand what God was up to, he had plenty of reason to believe that God was not being unjust, cruel, or unfair by allowing things in his life to crumble (Job 42).

    The apostle Paul experienced a physical problem that he attributed to Satan. He called it a "thorn in the flesh... , a messenger of Satan to buffet me," (2 Cor. 12:7). Paul prayed to have the thorn taken away, but God did not answer that prayer. Instead, He helped Paul to see how the difficulty could serve a good purpose. This weakness made Paul humbly dependent on God and put him in a position to experience God's grace (vv.8-10). [Although most cases of sickness cannot be directly tied to Satan's work, the gospel accounts do record a few examples of suffering attributed to Satan, including a blind and mute man (Matt. 12:22) and a boy who suffered seizures (17:14-18).]

- **God sometimes uses suffering to get our attention.** Some people turn away from God when they face difficulties, but for a number of people the suffering brings them into a closer relationship with God. Says Karen, a woman with lupus, "I decided that, regardless of my circumstances, I would much rather have God beside me than live my life without Him." In *Where Is God When It Hurts?*, author Philip Yancey writes about Joni Eareckson Tada, "She wrestled with God, yes, but she did not turn away from Him...Joni now calls her accident a 'glorious intruder,' and claims it was the best thing that ever happened to her. God used it to get her attention and direct her thoughts toward Him," (3).

    Paul wrote similar things about his physical troubles. The Lord told Paul, "My grace is sufficient for you, for My strength is made perfect in weakness," (2 Cor. 12:9). Then Paul added, "Therefore I take pleasure in infirmities, in reproaches, in needs, in persecutions, in distresses, for Christ's sake. For when I am weak, then I am strong," (v.10).

- **Suffering forces us to evaluate the direction of our lives.** We can choose to despair by focusing on our present problems, or we can choose to hope by recognizing God's long-range plan for us (Rom. 5:5; 8:18,28; Heb. 11). Suffering makes us recognize how weak the things that we put our faith in really are. Our finances, our jobs, our health, our loved ones, can all be taken away, and then what are we to depend on? By suffering, we are forced to reevaluate our priorities, values, goals, dreams, pleasures, the source of real strength, and our relationships with people and with God. If we don't turn away from God, it is bound to bring us into a closer relationship with God.

- **God suffers with us and is beside us in our darkest times.** Scripture assures us that He won't allow us to have more than we can handle.

- **Suffering puts us in the position where we need to be with other believers.** Paul uses the analogy of a human body (1 Cor. 12) to explain our need of other believers in order to function properly. "And if one member suffers, all the members suffer with it; or if one member is honored, all the members rejoice with it. Now you are the body of Christ, and members individually," (vv.26,27).

- **Suffering puts us in the position to bring comfort to others when they must suffer.** In 2 Corinthians 1, Paul writes, "Blessed be the God and Father of our Lord Jesus Christ, the Father of mercies and God of all comfort, who comforts us in all our tribulation, that we may be able to comfort those who are in any trouble, with the comfort with which we ourselves are comforted by God," (vv.3,4).

We cry out for complete answers. We feel abandoned in our suffering. Even Jesus Christ himself felt this way as he was hanging on the cross and cried out "My God! Why have you forsaken me?" We are not alone in our search for an explanation of our pain. Rather than give us an answer, God offers Himself to us instead. Through experience we learn that just knowing God is enough in order for us to live. If we know that we can trust Him, we don't need full explanations. We need to just rest in the peace that our pain and suffering are not meaningless. It's enough to know that God still rules the universe and that He really does care about us as individuals. John 14:27 says "The peace I give isn't like the peace the world gives. So don't be troubled or afraid." Just as we experience suffering that we do not understand, so too can we experience peace that is beyond human comprehension.

Yancey explains in *Where is God When it Hurts?* that the Bible doesn't always have an answer to our 'whys.'

> The Bible consistently changes the questions we bring to the problem of pain. It rarely, or ambiguously, answers the backward-looking question "Why?" Instead, it raises the very different, forward-looking question, "To what end?" We are not put on earth merely to satisfy our desires, to pursue life, liberty and happiness. We are here to be changed, to b made more like God in order to prepare us for a lifetime with him. And that process may be served by the mysterious pattern of all creation: pleasure sometimes emerges against a background of pain, evil may be transformed into good, and suffering may produce something of value (4).

When we begin to feel that God lacks concern about our pain, we need only look at the gift God gave us in sacrificing His son, Jesus Christ. God loved our suffering world so much that He sent His Son to agonize and die for us, to free us from being sentenced to eternal sorrow (John 3:16-18).

Chapter 7

Notes

Chapter 8
Where Do I Find Resources For My Group?

ESSENTIAL #8: *Finding Good Small Group Resources Makes a Difference*
In this chapter you will learn:
➤ *Where to find resources for your small group.*

Once you have decided to form a small group, you will likely start your search for materials. Unfortunately, you likely will not find an abundance of resources.

Rest Ministries, Inc. is pleased to let you know about *When Chronic Illness Enters Your Life*, a five lesson bible study for individuals or groups. A brief summary of the bible study follows:

Chronic illness is difficult.

There is no question... whether you have a deep relationship with Jesus Christ, or are just beginning to search for answers from Him, chronic illness can send you reeling into wondering "Where is God when it hurts?" and "Why do I have this illness?" Through these five bible studies you will:
- Learn how to feel God's presence when you feel so alone.
- Understand why God doesn't always give you the answers to your "whys."
- Find out how God can use you, even when you feel exhausted.
- Recognize ways to put your worries and fears about the future aside.
- Discover ways of building quality relationships, even when friends don't understand what you are going through.

Rest Ministries, Inc. also publishes a monthly support newsletter, *...And He Will Give You Rest.* Each issue features articles that address the emotional, relational, spiritual and practical issues of living with a chronic condition. Many articles in the newsletter could be helpful to lead group discussions.

Chapter 8

Examples of articles include:
- Patience! Is it Possible?
- Dealing with the Anger About Our Illness
- Spouses Speak Out About Their Feelings
- The Temptation of Comparison
- Our Changing Body Image
- What Has Knowing God Done For You Lately?

Each newsletter addresses the issues of illness in an upbeat and positive tone, while also discussing spirituality and offering encouragement.

Rest Ministries Comfort Zone Bookstore

Rest Ministries always has a great collection of books that address chronic illness, depression and more from a Christian perspective. Bibles studies, tapes a devotional book and more are examples of wonderful writing you will find here. Visit the bookstore online at www.comfortzonebooks.com or call or mail for a list of some current books and resources.

Resources

Be sure to sign up online for HopeNotes, the small group newsletter for HopeKeepers leaders where you will find additional resources and leadership ideas.

Here is a list of books that have been recommended as being excellent sources of information regarding chronic illness. Many of these may be useful tools for discussion in your group environment.

- *How to Help a Heartbroken Friend,* David Biebel. (1996, New Spire Publishing).
- *If God is so Good, Why do I Hurt So Bad?* David Biebel (1997, New Spire Publishing).
- *Pain: The Gift Nobody Wants,* Dr. Paul Brand & Philip Yancey. (1993, Harper Collins).
- *Anatomy of an Illness,* Norman Cousins. (1979, Bantam Books).
- *Sick and Tired of Feeling Sick and Tired,* Paul Donoghue and Mary Siegel. (1992, Norton and Company).
- *You Gotta Keep Dancing,* Tim Hansel. (1985, David C. Cook Publishing)
- *We Are Not Alone, Learning to Live with Chronic Illness,* Sefra Kobrin Pitzele. (1986, Thompson and Company).
- *Successful Living with Chronic Illness,* Kathleen Lewis. (1994, Kendall/Hunt Publishing).
- *When Life Becomes Precious: A Guide for Loved Ones and Friends of Cancer Patients,* Elise NeeDell Babcock. (1997, Bantam).
- *I Hurt Too Much for a Band-Aid,* Dr. Ken Olson. (1980, O'Sullivan Woodside & Co).
- *Where Is God When It Hurts?* Philip Yancey. (1977, Zondervan)

Chapter 9
Finding the need and filling it

ESSENTIAL #9: Only by Filling the Need Will Your Ministry Succeed
In this chapter you will learn:
➤ How to make your small group meeting accessible and comfortable.
➤ How to know what people want out of the small group.
➤ Some of the problems you may encounter with chronic illness/pain ministry.
➤ How to encourage people to come to small group meetings,

Now that you understand chronic illness/pain ministry, small group ministry, and you've got some materials for your group, you're ready to plan your goals for the group and get it going. Do you have any idea what people would like? What will make a chronic illness small group successful?

Make it Accessible and Comfortable

The first thing to do is to choose your meeting place.
⇒ Make it as conveniently located as possible. Although some people may be willing to drive over 15 miles if they hear wonderful things about the group, the closer it is to their home, the more likely they are to come.
⇒ Make sure there is enough parking. If you are having the meeting in a home, let people know what the parking situation will be like and be sensitive to how far people will have to park. If you live in an apartment and the visitor parking is at the back of the complex, do not have your home be your meeting place. People don't want to park far and walk around a complex looking for your apartment number. They will just go home.
⇒ Try to have chairs that are as comfortable as possible. Avoid straight back chairs or chairs that are especially low to the ground.
⇒ Set the room to a comfortable temperature. Don't try to freeze anyone out or turn up the heat. Usually 72-73 degrees Fahrenheit is comfortable.
⇒ Make sure bathrooms are accessible. If you are having the meeting in the home, make sure the bathroom is available without having to climb stairs. Check to make sure the toilet handle and sink faucet knobs can be easily be turned on and off.
⇒ Inform those who will be attending to avoid wearing colognes or perfumes to the meetings. Many people are sensitive to chemicals.
⇒ If you are serving drinks, make sure you have something available that is

decaffeinated. Have cold filtered water available. If you are serving snacks, stick with fresh fruit or vegetables and maybe a light dip. Many people may be watching their diet.

⇒ Give good directions and a map to anyone who will be attending for the first time. Add landmarks that can be seen in the dark.

Do not meet at your home if:
- You live more than 3-4 miles from the church.
- There is not enough parking.
- Available parking is more than 50 feet from your front door.
- You have more than 2 stairs to get into your home.
- There is not enough seating (don't expect people to sit on the floor.)
- Your only accessible bathroom is upstairs.
- You have pets that people could be allergic to.

If your church does not have a place where the group can meet, and your home is not a possibility, consider asking people in your church if they would be able to volunteer their home. You can also check into meeting at a public place, like a library or a restaurant; although these places will not offer the group as much privacy.

Choose a Date and Time

If people have already signed up for the small group, you may want to call around and get a consensus of when they would like to meet. You may find, however, that everyone has a different preference and this may be more trouble than it is worth. The best option is often to pick an evening, announce it, and have people RSVP so you know if the date/time will work.

Most people prefer to meet once a month, or possibly twice. Don't have your meetings run over two hours and make a point to end on time. People who are in pain will not want to stay out too late, they can't sit for long, and they were probably exhausted when they arrived, so respect their time.

Tackle the Topics People Want to Discuss

Now it's time for the fun stuff: the topic selection. At your first meeting you may want to have a 15-minute brainstorm session to have people list all of the topics they would like to see discussed in the future. This has a few benefits:
- People will be interested in returning if they know that these issues will be discussed in the future.
- People will feel like they will have some input to the group and they will be aware that the leader isn't going to be "preaching" all of the time.
- Discussing frustrations and fears will probably bring a few laughs, as everyone realizes that they aren't the only one feeling these feelings.

Here is a list from one brainstorming session:
- I would like to share my concerns about my future.
- I would like to talk about my family's future with my illness.

Chapter 9

- I need to find ways of dealing with my husband who can't acknowledge my illness.
- I need to express frustration about the relationships I have lost since I was diagnosed with an illness.
- I'd like to talk about how to cope with people who say you aren't healed because of lack of faith.
- I would like to talk about how to raise my kids while living with this illness. How do I make them understand that God isn't punishing me?
- I'd like to hear from others how they cope and how they've managed to 'get this far.'
- I'd like someone to cry with when the pain gets unbearable.
- The "Why me?" syndrome.
- I'd like to hear about how other people's marriages are affected by their illnesses and how they keep it positive.
- I'd like to discuss how I blame God for not healing me.
- I'd like to share experiences that are uplifting
- I'd like to talk about research and medical updates that improve all illnesses.
- Encouragement and hope to go on—how to find it in scripture.
- I'd like to discuss something that would increase my faith in God, in people, and myself; something that would keep my feet on the solid ground.
- I'd like to hear about when alternative medicines become too "new age." Where do we draw the line?
- I would like to hear how God has worked in others' lives through illness.

"The only thing that prevents me from going to church is when I am unable to drive safely, but I can usually get a ride. I have come to church vomiting (not the contagious of course). I have come to church in severe pain. I have found that if you are going to be sick anyway, you might as well make the most of it. After a year of bedrest, I am not crazy about staying home. I might as well be somewhere in the presence of worship than at home in bed. Sick is sick; It doesn't seem to matter to me where I am." — Jenny

"Maybe if the churches had a class just for sufferers, like they have the 'Singles' class or the 'Retired Adults.' We could each bring our experiences with pain, health care managers, spouses, children, worries, our troubles about getting around, loss and facing the inevitable 'end,' and share our ideas and concerns with each other. Just knowing there are others who deal with these things daily and can help one with coping, is a big step toward accepting all we must accept. Also, a class could help those who can't deal with the spiritual aspects of illness, such as the 'Why me-syndrome?' or blaming God for not healing them. It seems reasonable to me that we need to develop a 'place' of our own in our respective churches." — Lynette

"I think if I was to be motivated by anything it would be pure friendship and Godly love; Just a group of people who allow me to be me and no longer have to pretend. I'm tired of the mask." — Virginia

Chapter 9

When People Don't Come

The flyers go out announcing the beginning of the chronic pain ministry. And then the calls began.
- "I signed up for this because it sounded interesting, but I am in remission right now and I don't really feel like talking about my illness."
- "I'd really like to come, but I am so tired. I just can't make it tonight. Please forgive me."
- "I wish I could be there, but I really need to work late tonight since I had a doctor's appointment this morning and I went home early yesterday. I'll try to make the next meeting, I promise!"

The problem with chronic pain ministry is *everyone is in pain!* These factors are not shared with you to discourage you, but to let you be aware of some of the hurdles that you may encounter when you start your small group ministry.

- **People are stretched to the limits in time constraints.** If she is a parent, she is probably coping with the guilt of not being able to always participate in her child's activities. If an evening comes along and she feels good, chances are the parent is going to stay home and play. She doesn't know when she will feel good again, and the chronic pain group will always be there.

- **People have different limitations.** Some people will be able to get in the car, drive 15 minutes and sit through a two-hour meeting. Others will not. Some will be able to do it easily. For some, it will take an enormous amount of energy to get there are participate. Everyone has his or her individual limitations.

- **People have their own body clocks.** Some people get up early in the morning and get as much done as they can because after noon their energy starts dissipating. Others will just be climbing out of bed at noon, and will finally be able to walk around by 5 p.m. You have the challenge of finding a meeting time that will best suit everyone who would like to attend.

- **People have different responsibilities.** Some people will work full-time, some will work part-time and some won't work at all. Again, finding a meeting time that works for as many people as possible may be a challenge, but it is possible!

- **People who aren't currently in pain, won't want to come.** Who wants to think about pain any more than they must? You'll find that when people start to feel good, they won't want to come. Accept this and keep in touch with them, because chances are, at some point, they will want and need your support again.

Chapter 9

Things That Will Encourage People to Come

Small group leaders who are involved with chronic illness/pain ministry contributed a few of their ideas about what makes a small group effective.

- Open it up to people outside of your church. Although you may want to have it be a ministry of your church, encourage people outside of your church to attend as well. Oftentimes, a chronic illness/pain group will meet a need and a person will come to the church *because* of this.

- Put up flyers about your ministry at local Christian bookstores, Christian coffeehouses, etc. Find creative ways of advertising your ministry so that people know it exists.

- Set up a meeting time that is consistent, such as "the first Tuesday of the month" so people always know when the meeting is and can plan on it each month.

- Invite speakers to come and lead a discussion on a variety of topics. For example, people will relate to a Christian who is a physical therapist, as well as be encouraged to be reminded of the Christians in the medical field.

- Have people share what they have learned through their illness journey and how they came to this point. Provide inspirational messages from others. Encourage people to keep a journal and then share what they would like from it.

- Include the topic of your next speaker in the church bulletin. People who may not currently be in pain may be encouraged to come and hear the presenter anyway.

- Beware of spending too much time talking about potential treatments and alternative medicine. Many people are looking for a refuge away from that. If people wish to discuss their treatments, encourage them to do so after the meeting.

- Respect people's time. Make sure that the meeting has breaks to get up and stretch and that you end on time.

- Invite spouses or loved ones to some of the meetings and encourage them to communicate with one another about their challenges, blessings, etc.

- Make sure people in church leadership are aware of the small group, so that when they talk to someone who has a chronic illness, they can inform them of your small group.

Some chronic illness small groups work very well and others seem to have some trouble getting off of the ground. Don't feel discouraged if your group is taking time to form, but stick with it. Over time, people will come to depend on it and look forward to finding a place of refuge where they can opening discuss their illness and their spiritual journey.

If you have questions about forming a chronic illness/pain small group in your church or community, Lisa Copen, founder of Rest Ministries, Inc. *is available to discuss it with you and lead you through the process. A HopeKeepers Start Up Kit is also available if your church is interested in an entire package of materials to start the group off for about $300.*
Call 888-751-7378.

25 Ways to Publicize Your Group

Within the church:

1. Have your group listed in the small group section of your church resource list.
2. Request a special blurb in the church bulletin on Sunday about the HK group.
3. Propose an article for your church newsletter about your experience living with chronic illness and at the end encourage others to come to the HK group.
4. If possible, ask the church leaders if you can get up at church and personally announce the ministry and why you feel God has led you on this path.
5. Make a list up of all of the reasons that people don't come and then write down a way that you can address this. Remember this from your HK info packet? "I'd like to start a HopeKeepers group but…"
6. Are there people who you think may benefit but they don't think they need it, especially elderly? Ask them if they would consider being on a 3-5 person panel and sharing with "younger folk" about how they've lived successfully with illness and what they would give as advice for those tough times.
7. If your church has a ministry faire, be sure to have a table with brochures and newsletters to distribute. Rest Ministries will gladly send you materials to distribute.
8. Ask your church who it is that visits people in the hospital, etc. and explain to them about HopeKeepers. Give them some copies of the newsletters that they can pass on if they feel appropriate and let the church leader know that HopeKeepers is there when the person leaves the hospital if s/he feels up to joining in.
9. Plan an evening with spouses and ask everyone to be prepared to talk about one challenge that they have had and one lesson that they have learned.
10. Ask your church if you can always have brochures available on the resource table. Rest Ministries has brochures "When a Friend has a Chronic Illness: What to Say, How to Help" and church attendees love these.
11. If people have signed up for the group, but they aren't dedicated to getting there, begin by having you and a friend write notes of encouragement to them, reminding them that you care whether they come or not. They just may start showing up!
12. Mention the existence and the need of the group to other church leaders. Many of their families will have illness and even if they feel it doesn't meet their needs, it may of someone that they know. Inform the women and men's minis-

try leaders so when people talk to them about their troubles, they can refer them to your group.
13. Also inform the local doctors, nurses, counselors, etc. that attend your church.

Outside of the church: (with church approval)

1. Call local churches and hospitals and let them know that you have a HK group and that it is open for others to attend. Rest Ministries can provide brochures or call them if they have questions.
2. Put an add in your local papers, either secular or Christian. Skim through the whole paper. It may be able to be listed under health, religion, elderly, caregiving, etc.
3. Send a letter to your local paper and include any photos. For an example press release see ours (it's a bit long, but it's our "general" one for the web) at http://www.restministries.org/admin-media.htm
4. Place brochures at your local hospital or doctors office with permission.
5. Mention HK to your physicians and let them know that others are welcome. Oftentimes doctors are glad to hear that you are doing positive things despite your illness.
6. Read the newspapers and whenever there is an article about some similar group, call them and tell them about your own. Connect with others. Also, keep track of the reporters that do these stories. Writers will often do similar styles of articles in the future.
7. Pay attention to specific dates and use these to boost your group at local events or to make an announcement at church. Oct. is national disability awareness month, Nov. is national caregiver's month, May in national fibromyalgia awareness month. Simply the timing can make your group newsworthy!
8. If you have a local Christian radio show send them a brochure and some information on how HK is needed and see if you can get on as a guest. It may seem a bit scary at first but God will get you through it!
9. Post flyers with tear-offs of your phone number at local health clubs, rehabilitation clinics or senior centers where people may be looking at the bulletin boards.
10. Exhibit at local health fairs, cancer runs, etc. If you explain that you are nonprofit and not selling anything they will often give you complimentary booth space and you will get to meet a lot of people. Get help! Don't try to do it on your own. Whenever you hear about a local event in your area that you cannot attend or exhibit at, call to see if they have a general resource table and if you could have some brochures available.
11. Call Lisa at Rest Ministries and ask that we do a mailing of postcards to people in your area about your group. Send or email us the information and we will take care of the rest and invite people from our mailing list.
12. Talk a lot. Get a Rest Ministries T-Shirt. Ask Lisa about our Verse cards (much better than a business card!) and carry them with you. Whenever people ask about your illness turn the conversation around to what God is teaching you through it and how he's working in your HopeKeepers

group and then give them a verse card that they can pass on. With 1 in 3 people living with a chronic condition in the US, everyone knows a few people who could use a boost. And if they aren't in your area, connect them with Rest Ministries and we will make sure they connect with a HopeKeepers group somewhere!

Don't forget to participate in National Invisible Chronic Illness Awareness Week held annually the last week of September and sponsored by Rest Ministries, Inc.

www.invisibleillness.com

Chapter 10
How to Keep the Chronic Illness-Pain Ministry in the Forefront

ESSENTIAL #10: Chronic Illness Is Invisible

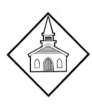

Essential #10 may sound familiar, because it was essential #1 as well. *Chronic illness and pain are invisible.* As you have began to form a chronic illness/pain ministry you have probably answered a lot of questions. People have said, "I didn't even know you had a chronic illness. You look so good!" Church leadership may have asked, "Why do we need a ministry for people with chronic illness? If God hasn't healed them, we shouldn't condone their sin by offering them a group." Perhaps when you announced your small group, you had few people sign up and others said, "There just isn't that great of a need."

Don't believe them. There are large numbers of people who are hurting, and they feel invisible. They may not always be quick to respond to a group, because they worry about becoming vulnerable. They may feel they just don't have the time. You may be excited about new bible study materials that you have found, but no one else is. Don't despair. Remember, people don't care how much you know until they know how much you care. Chronic illness/pain ministry takes time. It takes times to develop friendships. It takes time for people to trust you. It takes time for them to see your motivations for leading a chronic illness/pain small group. They want to see that you are sincere and not just another body that the church has sent over to their house to feel sorry for them and give them advice. Give it time.

In the meantime, focus your energies on developing the entire chronic illness/pain ministry, not just the small group.
- Ask the church leadership if you could come into their office one day and explain your experiences with living with chronic illness and how this group of people could be better ministered to.
- Take time to find quality, sincere volunteers who want to be a part of a ministry that will make a difference.
- Put up flyers about your small group meetings in community locations.
- Plan a picnic for people who live with chronic illness/pain (and have it

catered to motivate them to comer!) Let people know it will be fun, not a depressing afternoon.

All of these are ways in which your chronic illness ministry can be visible. There will be many people in your church who live with illness who will be watching the ministry to see what it is like. They want to know if it will truly be a refuge, or if every meeting will include a healing ceremony. They will want to know if the meetings are going to include discussion of alternative medicines. They are waiting and watching. So now is the time to truly let everyone know what you stand for, and in time, your participation level will improve.

In 2002, Rest Ministries began National Invisible Chronic Illness Awareness Week during the last week of September. This week is an opportunity for the public to be informed about those who live with invisible disabilities. Churches are encouraged to participate in ways such as (1) Having brochures available "When a Friend Has a Chronic Illness: What to Say, How to Help"; (2) Have the pastor do a sermon on chronic pain or illness, or even suffering; (3) Volunteer to give your testimony about how God has worked through your illness to mold you into who He desires you to be; (4) Kick off your HopeKeepers meeting in September.

Many individuals put up posters, do radio and television interviews, hand out brochures and more. For more information or to find out about being a sponsor see www.invisibleillness.com .

Rest Ministries uses this week as a chance to educate the public about invisible illness, but even more so as a way to reach out to those who are hurting and share with them the hope found in Jesus.

Conclusion

If you do not live with illness or pain, I hope this book has given you the opportunity to look inside the world of the chronically ill. You may have said, "Hmm...I never knew that," or "I never thought of that, but it makes sense."

If you live with illness or pain, I hope that you have been able to nod in agreement and feel as though someone has finally said what you knew all along. I hope that you have thought, "I'm not alone."

Many people have shared their opinions throughout this book and it would not have been nearly as effective without their participation, as they recalled their personal experience. Whether you have an illness or not, I hope that their comments have made an impact on you. When I started writing this book, I had some assumptions that the church was not doing all that it could to outreach to people who live with illness or pain. Unfortunately, the many comments I received proved that this was true, and in some instances, it was bitterly accurate. Over and over, people poured out their frustrations, their disappointments, and their hurts, some of which had been carried for years.

We understand that we cannot expect the church to be perfect and meet every need that we have, but we do expect that it should be a place where we will not be judged, condemned, or chastised. To be fair, some people shared that they were pleased with how their church has responded to their illness, but these were by far the minority.

Yancey shares in *Where is God When it Hurts?*,
> "The French have a saying: 'To suffer passes; to have suffered never passes.' Too often we think about a ministry of helps as a one-way street in which I, the healthy person, reach out in compassion to assist the wounded. But people who have suffered are the very best equipped to help, and a person crosses the final barrier of helplessness when he or she learns to use the experience of suffering itself as a means of reaching out to others...A wise sufferer will look not inward, but outward. There is no more effective healer than a wounded healer, and in the process the wounded healer's own scars may fade away." [1]

I hope that you can be a wounded healer.

> *"Come and let us return to the Lord, for He has torn us so that he may heal us; He has stricken so that He may bind us up."*
> Hosea 6:1

---

1   Yancey, Philip. *Where Is God When It Hurts?* 1977, Zondervan. p. 193.

Your Comments

We are always interested in hearing from you! Whether you would like to share your story or sorrows, we read each letter. Your comments help us shape the ministry and direct the newsletter articles and bible studies to be what you are looking for. With your permission, your comments may be included. Please include:
- your name
- your address
- is permission granted to quote you? (first names used only)

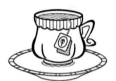

Rest Ministries, Inc.
serving people who live with chronic illness or pain.

Rest Ministries, Inc. is a non-profit service ministry whose purpose is to serve people who live with chronic illness or pain, and their families, by providing spiritual, emotional, relational and practical support through a variety of resources, including a monthly newsletter, bible studies, and small group materials. We also seek to bring an awareness and a change in action throughout churches in the U.S. in regard to how people who live with chronic illness/pain are served, and teach churches effective ministry tools to outreach to this population.

Rest Ministries, Inc. features a monthly newsletter, ...*And He Will Give You Rest,* that is heartening and uplifting. As well as offering practical information and available resources, it addresses needs that people in chronic pain have that the medical field rarely takes time to acknowledge. For example, how to explain to others how you are feeling, how to get your grocery shopping done when you are exhausted, and feedback from spouses of people in pain. ...*And He Will Give You Rest* also speaks to the spiritual side of the person in chronic pain, featuring articles such as *How God Can Work Through Your Exhaustion, Finding the Comfort Zone With Family and Friends,* a monthly devotional and informational web sites.

> *"Rest Ministries, Inc. fills a void in health care for those dealing with chronic illness. It is a source of inspiration and hope for anyone who is coping with difficult times. The newsletter's topics give comfort to those in need in an easy-to-read format. I recommend it enthusiastically."*
> —Elise NeeDell Babcock, author of *When Life Becomes Precious* (Bantam, 1997) and founder of Cancer Counseling, Inc.

Be sure to check us out on the web!
http://www.restministries.org

Ordering Information

shipping is included in all prices

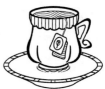

- ...*And He Will Give You Rest* newsletter
  1 year subscription (12 issues) $15.00   _____
  2 year subscription (24 issues) $28.00   _____
  Foreign   (12 issues) $24 US funds   _____
- Be a HopeKeeper: Includes 12 issues of *And He Will Give You Rest*, 1 copy of When Chronic Illness Enters Your Life and early-bird discounts on new materials. $25   _____
- Mosaic Moments Devotional $ 12.00   _____
- A Woman's Health Resource Journal $28.95   _____
- *So You Want to Start a Chronic Illness/Pain Ministry: 10 Essentials For Making it Work* $14.50   _____

Bible studies
- *When Chronic Illness* Enters Your Life $6.50   _____
- *Learning to Live with Chronic Illness* $6.50   _____

❏ I would like to make a gift to *Rest Ministries* in the amount of _____
❏ I would like to partner with *Rest Ministries* & I pledge to give _____ each month.
   * Rest Ministries, Inc. is a 501(c)(3) nonprofit. Your gift is tax-deductible.
❏ I am interested in starting a HopeKeeper Group for people who live with chronic illness or pain. Please send me a HopeKeepers information packet.
❏ I would like information about a devotional for people who live with chronic illness or pain.
   TOTAL Purchases/Gifts: $ _____

California residents add 7.75% to T-shirt purchase $ _____

TOTAL: $ _____

Include check made payable to Rest Ministries
Charge my: ❏ **Visa**   ❏ **Mastercard**
Card # _____
Expiration date:_____
Cardholder's signature *(required)* _____

Send to: Rest Ministries, Inc.
                   P.O Box 502928, San Diego, CA 92150

Name:_____

Address: _____

City/State/Zip_____

Phone number:_____

Email _____

Gifts

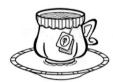

As a non-profit ministry, we are always grateful for any tax-deductible monetary donations that we receive. We are currently funded solely by donations. Your donation will be used to provide:

- Ongoing encouragement to people who live with chronic illness in the forms of a monthly support newsletter and other resources and programs.
- The ability to form *HopeKeepers* small groups for people who live with illness or pain and support materials.
- The opportunity for us to continue to reach out to churches, educating them on how to better serve

Name_____

Address_____

Phone number _____

I would like to make a donation to assist *Rest Ministries, Inc.* with encouraging more people, developing materials for people who live with pain, forming *HopeKeepers* small groups, and teaching churches how to serve those who live with chronic illness or pain.

_____ $25 _____ $250
_____ $50 _____ $500
_____ $100 _____ $1000
_____ $150 Other_____

Make check payable to: Rest Ministries
Send to: Rest Ministries, Inc.
P.O. Box 502928
San Diego, CA 92150

Rest Ministries, Inc. is a non-profit 501(c)3 organization. Your gift is tax-deductable.

Notes

A Devotional Book From Rest Ministries

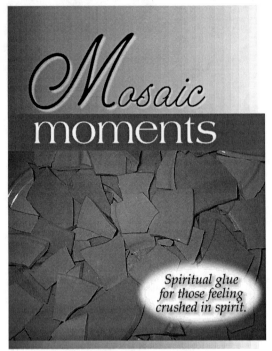

Devotionals for the Chronically Ill
LISA J. COPEN

Over 20 Contributors!

"There are times when chronic illness threatens to steal something new from every area of life. It is then that Rest Ministries has proven to be my lifeline, their daily devotionals I receive via e-mail providing manna for the moment. *Mosaic Moments* has stocked that manna in a single comforting compilation. A virtual cupboard brimming with heart-to-heart stories grounded in Biblical truth, it is written by real people in the trenches of chronic illness... people who deal with the very issues I face each day as I live with chronic pain caused by neurofibromatosis. I finished each serving not simply fulfilled, but encouraged to go on. *Mosaic Moments* is truly heaven's *Chicken Soup for the Chronically Ill Soul*." Roberta Messner, PhD, RN, *author of numerous medical and inspirational articles on living with chronic pain; Contributor to* Guideposts *and* Daily Guideposts.

"These devotions are not empty morsels *promising* nutrition, but *real* meat from the Life Giver Himself for those so desperately needing spiritual sustenance. May God bless your work." Darlene K. Hanson, *Librarian for Polio Experience Network and a Horizon Hospice volunteer*

"*Mosaic Moments* illustrates what people with hidden illnesses are becoming in the hands of God's workmanship. I must confess that their spiritual development, maturity and insight are far ahead of mine." Don Crooker *President of the Christian Council on Persons with Disabilities, Int.*

"I am so thankful to be able to offer *Mosaic Moments* as a resource to those who struggle with chronic pain and illness. Rarely are there words to convey my heartfelt concerns for suffering. With *Mosaic Moments* I am able to share a spiritual cup of cold water. It offers words of loving and caring I believe Jesus Himself would share." Julie Russell, *R.N., Parish Nurse, Stephen Minister*

"It's amazing! So many U-turns in this world involve the work of God's hand through illness, but it's often hard to see the end result when you are in pain. *Mosaic Moments* is a daily guidepost for those who are suffering, offering compassion, understanding, joy and even humor. Lisa and others become vulnerable to give a glimpse into their journey and what sustains them." Allison Gappa Bottke, *author of* God Allows U-Turns *series.*

"The authors of *Mosaic Moments* prove that just because you have pain doesn't mean you have to be one. With joy flooding forth in concise bursts of truth and integrity, they write convincingly and hopefully. This book is written by those who know for those who know." Phillip H. Barnhart, *Doctor of Ministry, Founding Pastor and Pastor Emeritus of Chapel on the Hill, Lake Geneva, Wisconsin*

Just $12 includes shipping.
Order at Rest Ministries web site
www.comfortzonebooks.com
888-751-7378